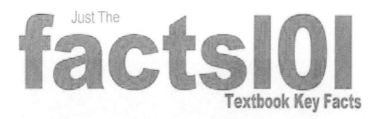

Just The

facts101
Textbook Key Facts

Textbook Outlines, Highlights, and Practice Quizzes

Health Promotion Throughout the Life Span

by Carole Lium Edelman, 7th Edition

All "Just the Facts101" Material Written or Prepared by Cram101 Publishing

Title Page

Visit Cram101.com for full Practice Exams

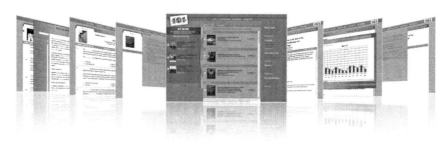

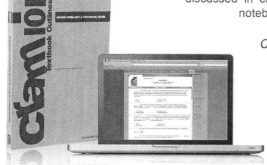

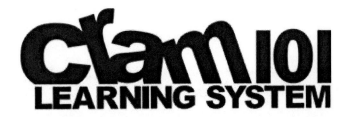

"Just the Facts101" is a Cram101 publication and tool designed to give you all the facts from your textbooks. Visit Cram101.com for the full practice test for each of your chapters for virtually any of your textbooks.

Cram101 has built custom study tools specific to your textbook. We provide all of the factual testable information and unlike traditional study guides, we will never send you back to your textbook for more information.

YOU WILL NEVER HAVE TO HIGHLIGHT A BOOK AGAIN!

Cram101 StudyGuides

All of the information in this StudyGuide is written specifically for your textbook. We include the key terms, places, people, and concepts... the information you can expect on your next exam!

Want to take a practice test?

Throughout each chapter of this StudyGuide you will find links to cram101.com where you can select specific chapters to take a complete test on, or you can subscribe and get practice tests for up to 12 of your textbooks, along with other exclusive cram101.com tools like problem solving labs and reference libraries.

Cram101.com

Only cram101.com gives you the outlines, highlights, and PRACTICE TESTS specific to your textbook. Cram101.com is an online application where you'll discover study tools designed to make the most of your limited study time.

By purchasing this book, you get 50% off the normal subscription free!. Just enter the promotional code **'DK73DW20273'** on the Cram101.com registration screen.

www.Cram101.com

Learning System

facts101

Health Promotion Throughout the Life Span
Carole Lium Edelman, 7th

CONTENTS

Chapter 1. Health Defined: Objectives for Promotion and Prevention,

_____ Alternative medicine

_____ Weight loss

_____ Primary care

_____ Sick role

_____ Health care

_____ Health education

_____ Public health

_____ World Health Organization

_____ Population health

_____ Toilet training

_____ Health disparities

_____ Cultural competence

_____ Problem solving

_____ Health promotion

_____ Life expectancy

_____ Case study

_____ Transtheoretical model

_____ Nursing

_____ Risk factor

Trisomy

CHAPTER HIGHLIGHTS & NOTES: KEY TERMS, PEOPLE, PLACES, CONCEPTS

Alternative medicine	In Western culture, Alternative medicine is any healing practice 'that does not fall within the realm of conventional medicine', or 'that which has not been shown consistently to be effective.' It is often opposed to evidence based medicine and encompasses therapies with an historical or cultural, rather than a scientific, basis. The American National Center for Complementary and Alternative medicine cites examples including naturopathy, chiropractic, herbalism, traditional Chinese medicine, Ayurveda, meditation, yoga, biofeedback, hypnosis, homeopathy, acupuncture, and nutritional-based therapies, in addition to a range of other practices. It is frequently grouped with complementary medicine, which generally refers to the same interventions when used in conjunction with mainstream techniques, under the umbrella term complementary and Alternative medicine, or CAM.
Weight loss	Weight loss, in the context of medicine, health or physical fitness, is a reduction of the total body mass, due to a mean loss of fluid, body fat or adipose tissue and/or lean mass, namely bone mineral deposits, muscle, tendon and other connective tissue. It can occur unintentionally due to an underlying disease or can arise from a conscious effort to improve an actual or perceived overweight or obese state. Unintentional weight loss Unintentional weight loss occurs in many diseases and conditions, including some very serious diseases such as cancer, AIDS, and a variety of other diseases.
Primary care	Primary care is a term used for the activity of a health care provider who acts as a first point of consultation for all patients. Continuity of care is also a key characteristic of Primary care. Primary care is an important form of health access for patients.
Sick role	Sick role is a term used in medical sociology concerning the social aspects of falling ill and the privileges and obligations that accompany it. It is a concept created by American sociologist Talcott Parsons in 1951.

Health care	Health care , refers to the treatment and management of illness, and the preservation of health through services offered by the medical, dental, complementary and alternative medicine, pharmaceutical, clinical laboratory sciences , nursing, and allied health professions. Health care embraces all the goods and services designed to promote health, including 'preventive, curative and palliative interventions, whether directed to individuals or to populations'. Before the term Health care became popular, English-speakers referred to medicine or to the health sector and spoke of the treatment and prevention of illness and disease.
Health education	Health education is the profession of educating people about health. Areas within this profession encompass environmental health, physical health, social health, emotional health, intellectual health, and spiritual health. It can be defined as the principle by which individuals and groups of people learn to behave in a manner conducive to the promotion, maintenance, or restoration of health.
Public health	Public health is 'the science and art of preventing disease, prolonging life and promoting health through the organized efforts and informed choices of society, organizations, public and private, communities and individuals.' (1920, C.E.A. Winslow) It is concerned with threats to the overall health of a community based on population health analysis. The population in question can be as small as a handful of people or as large as all the inhabitants of several continents (for instance, in the case of a pandemic). Public health is typically divided into epidemiology, biostatistics and health services.
World Health Organization	The World Health Organization is a specialized agency of the United Nations (UN) that acts as a coordinating authority on international public health. Established on 7 April 1948, and headquartered in Geneva, Switzerland, the agency inherited the mandate and resources of its predecessor, the Health Organization, which had been an agency of the League of Nations. The World Health Organization's constitution states that its objective 'is the attainment by all peoples of the highest possible level of health .' Its major task is to combat disease, especially key infectious diseases, and to promote the general health of the people of the world.
Population health	Population health has been defined as 'the health outcomes of a group of individuals, including the distribution of such outcomes within the group.' It is an approach to health that aims to improve the health of an entire population. One major step in achieving this aim is to reduce health inequities among population groups. Population health seeks to step beyond the individual-level focus of mainstream medicine and public health by addressing a broad range of factors that impact health on a population-level, such as environment, social structure, resource distribution, etc.

Chapter 1. Health Defined: Objectives for Promotion and Prevention,

CHAPTER HIGHLIGHTS & NOTES: KEY TERMS, PEOPLE, PLACES, CONCEPTS

Toilet training	Toilet training, or potty training, is the process of training a young child to use the toilet for urination and defecation, though training may start with a smaller toilet bowl-shaped device (often known as a potty). In Western countries it is usually started and completed between the ages of 12 months and three years with boys typically being at the higher end of the age spectrum. Cultural factors play a large part in what age is deemed appropriate, with the age being generally later in America. Most advise that Toilet training is a mutual task, requiring cooperation, agreement and understanding between child and the caregiver, and the best potty training techniques emphasize consistency and positive reinforcement over punishment - making it fun for the child.
Health disparities	Health disparities refer to gaps in the quality of health and health care across racial, ethnic, sexual orientation and socioeconomic groups. The Health Resources and Services Administration defines Health disparities as 'population-specific differences in the presence of disease, health outcomes, or access to health care.' In the United States, Health disparities are well documented in minority populations such as African Americans, Native Americans, Asian Americans, and Latinos. When compared to whites, these minority groups have higher incidence of chronic diseases, higher mortality, and poorer health outcomes.
Cultural competence	Cultural competence refers to an ability to interact effectively with people of different cultures. Cultural competence comprises four components: (a) Awareness of one's own cultural worldview, (b) Attitude towards cultural differences, (c) Knowledge of different cultural practices and worldviews, and (d) cross-cultural skills. Developing Cultural competence results in an ability to understand, communicate with, and effectively interact with people across cultures.
Problem solving	Problem solving is a mental process and is part of the larger problem process that includes problem finding and problem shaping. Considered the most complex of all intellectual functions, Problem solving has been defined as higher-order cognitive process that requires the modulation and control of more routine or fundamental skills. Problem solving occurs when an organism or an artificial intelligence system needs to move from a given state to a desired goal state.
Health promotion	Health promotion has been defined by the World Health Organization's 2005 Bangkok Charter for Health promotion in a Globalized World as 'the process of enabling people to increase control over their health and its determinants, and thereby improve their health'.

Visit Cram101.com for full Practice Exams

	The primary means of Health promotion occur through developing healthy public policy that addresses the prerequisites of health such as income, housing, food security, employment, and quality working conditions. There is a tendency among public health officials and governments -- and this is especially the case in liberal nations such as Canada and the USA -- to reduce Health promotion to health education and social marketing focused on changing behavioral risk factors.
Life expectancy	Life expectancy is the average number of years of life remaining at a given age. The term is most often used in the human context, but used also in plant or animal ecology and the calculation is based on the analysis of life tables (also known as actuarial tables). The term may also be used in the context of manufactured objects although the related term shelf life is used for consumer products and the term mean time to breakdown (MTTB) is used in engineering literature.
Case study	A Case study is a research methodology common in social science. It is based on an in-depth investigation of a single individual, group, or event to explore causation in order to find underlying principles.
Transtheoretical model	The Transtheoretical model in health psychology is intended to explain or predict a person's success or failure in achieving a proposed behavior change, such as developing different habits. It attempts to answer why the change 'stuck' or alternatively why the change was not made. The Transtheoretical model is also known by the acronym 'TTranstheoretical model' and by the term 'stages of change model'.
Nursing	Nursing is a healthcare profession focused on the care of individuals, families, and communities so they may attain, maintain, or recover optimal health and quality of life from conception to death. Nurses work in a large variety of specialties where they work independently and as part of a team to assess, plan, implement and evaluate care. Nursing Science is a field of knowledge based on the contributions of nursing scientist through peer reviewed scholarly journals and evidenced-based practice.
Risk factor	A Risk factor is a variable associated with an increased risk of disease or infection. Risk factors are correlational and not necessarily causal, because correlation does not imply causation. For example, being young cannot be said to cause measles, but young people are more at risk as they are less likely to have developed immunity during a previous epidemic.
Trisomy	A Trisomy is a genetic abnormality in which there are three copies, instead of the normal two, of a particular chromosome.

Visit Cram101.com for full Practice Exams

Chapter 1. Health Defined: Objectives for Promotion and Prevention,

A Trisomy is a type of aneuploidy (an abnormal number of chromosomes).

Most organisms that reproduce sexually have pairs of chromosomes in each cell, with one chromosome inherited from each parent.

CHAPTER QUIZ: KEY TERMS, PEOPLE, PLACES, CONCEPTS

1. _____ is 'the science and art of preventing disease, prolonging life and promoting health through the organized efforts and informed choices of society, organizations, public and private, communities and individuals.' (1920, C.E.A. Winslow) It is concerned with threats to the overall health of a community based on population health analysis. The population in question can be as small as a handful of people or as large as all the inhabitants of several continents (for instance, in the case of a pandemic). _____ is typically divided into epidemiology, biostatistics and health services.

   a. Public health
   b. Malnutrition
   c. Bacteriophage
   d. Baroreflex

2. _____, in the context of medicine, health or physical fitness, is a reduction of the total body mass, due to a mean loss of fluid, body fat or adipose tissue and/or lean mass, namely bone mineral deposits, muscle, tendon and other connective tissue. It can occur unintentionally due to an underlying disease or can arise from a conscious effort to improve an actual or perceived overweight or obese state.

   Unintentional _____

   Unintentional _____ occurs in many diseases and conditions, including some very serious diseases such as cancer, AIDS, and a variety of other diseases.

   a. abdominal exam
   b. Achilles tendon
   c. Acute HIV infection
   d. Weight loss

3. . In Western culture, _____ is any healing practice 'that does not fall within the realm of conventional medicine', or 'that which has not been shown consistently to be effective.' It is often opposed to evidence based medicine and encompasses therapies with an historical or cultural, rather than a scientific, basis. The American National Center for Complementary and _____ cites examples including naturopathy, chiropractic, herbalism, traditional Chinese medicine, Ayurveda, meditation, yoga, biofeedback, hypnosis, homeopathy, acupuncture, and nutritional-based therapies, in addition to a range of other practices. It is frequently grouped with complementary medicine, which generally refers to the same interventions when used in conjunction with mainstream techniques, under the umbrella term complementary and _____, or CAM.

a. abdominal exam
b. Achilles tendon
c. Acute HIV infection
d. Alternative medicine

4. The _____ in health psychology is intended to explain or predict a person's success or failure in achieving a proposed behavior change, such as developing different habits. It attempts to answer why the change 'stuck' or alternatively why the change was not made.

   The _____ is also known by the acronym 'TTranstheoretical model' and by the term 'stages of change model'.

   a. Transtheoretical model
   b. Baroreflex
   c. Benign prostatic hyperplasia
   d. Haven Institute

5. _____ is the profession of educating people about health. Areas within this profession encompass environmental health, physical health, social health, emotional health, intellectual health, and spiritual health. It can be defined as the principle by which individuals and groups of people learn to behave in a manner conducive to the promotion, maintenance, or restoration of health.

   a. Mahatma Gandhi Institute of Medical Sciences
   b. Health education
   c. Breastfeeding
   d. Mark Lester

1. a
2. d
3. d
4. a
5. b

You can take the complete Chapter Practice Test

for Chapter 1. Health Defined: Objectives for Promotion and Prevention,
on all key terms, persons, places, and concepts.

Online 99 Cents

http://www.epub1625.32.20273.1.cram101.com/

Use www.Cram101.com for all your study needs

including Cram101's online interactive problem solving labs in

chemistry, statistics, mathematics, and more.

Chapter 2. Emerging Populations and Health,

_____ Harm reduction

_____ Health education

_____ Mortality rate

_____ Toilet training

_____ Health system

_____ Mental health

_____ Health care

_____ Breast cancer

_____ Folk medicine

_____ Therapeutic touch

_____ Cardiovascular disease

_____ Health insurance

_____ Population health

_____ Lead poisoning

_____ Maternal death

_____ Prenatal care

_____ Blood pressure

_____ Alcohol abuse

_____ Medicine Man

CHAPTER OUTLINE: KEY TERMS, PEOPLE, PLACES, CONCEPTS

	Case study
	Community health
	Ambulatory care

CHAPTER HIGHLIGHTS & NOTES: KEY TERMS, PEOPLE, PLACES, CONCEPTS

| Harm reduction | Harm reduction refers to a range of pragmatic and evidence-based public health policies designed to reduce the harmful consequences associated with drug use and other high risk activities .

Many advocates argue that prohibitionist laws criminalize people for suffering from a disease and cause harm, for example by obliging drug addicts to obtain drugs of unknown purity from unreliable criminal sources at high prices, increasing the risk of overdose and death. . |
| --- | --- |
| Health education | Health education is the profession of educating people about health. Areas within this profession encompass environmental health, physical health, social health, emotional health, intellectual health, and spiritual health. It can be defined as the principle by which individuals and groups of people learn to behave in a manner conducive to the promotion, maintenance, or restoration of health. |
| Mortality rate | Mortality rate is a measure of the number of deaths (in general,) in some population, scaled to the size of that population, per unit time. Mortality rate is typically expressed in units of deaths per 1000 individuals per year; thus, a Mortality rate of 9.5 in a population of 100,000 would mean 950 deaths per year in that entire population. It is distinct from morbidity rate, which refers to the number of individuals in poor health during a given time period (the prevalence rate) or the number who currently have that disease (the incidence rate), scaled to the size of the population. |
| Toilet training | Toilet training, or potty training, is the process of training a young child to use the toilet for urination and defecation, though training may start with a smaller toilet bowl-shaped device (often known as a potty). In Western countries it is usually started and completed between the ages of 12 months and three years with boys typically being at the higher end of the age spectrum. |

Cultural factors play a large part in what age is deemed appropriate, with the age being generally later in America.

Most advise that Toilet training is a mutual task, requiring cooperation, agreement and understanding between child and the caregiver, and the best potty training techniques emphasize consistency and positive reinforcement over punishment - making it fun for the child.

Health system	A Health System can be defined as the structured and interrelated set of all actors and institutions contributing to health improvement. The health system boundaries could then be referred to the concept of health action, which is 'any set of activities whose primary intent is to improve or maintain health' . A wide concept Too often health systems have been defined with a reductionist perspective, for example reducing it to the health care systems.
Mental health	Mental health is a term used to describe either a level of cognitive or emotional well-being or an absence of a mental disorder. From perspectives of the discipline of positive psychology or holism Mental health may include an individual's ability to enjoy life and procure a balance between life activities and efforts to achieve psychological resilience. The World Health Organization defines Mental health as 'a state of well-being in which the individual realizes his or her own abilities, can cope with the normal stresses of life, can work productively and fruitfully, and is able to make a contribution to his or her community'.
Health care	Health care , refers to the treatment and management of illness, and the preservation of health through services offered by the medical, dental, complementary and alternative medicine, pharmaceutical, clinical laboratory sciences , nursing, and allied health professions. Health care embraces all the goods and services designed to promote health, including 'preventive, curative and palliative interventions, whether directed to individuals or to populations'. Before the term Health care became popular, English-speakers referred to medicine or to the health sector and spoke of the treatment and prevention of illness and disease.
Breast cancer	Breast cancer is cancer originating from breast tissue, most commonly from the inner lining of milk ducts or the lobules that supply the ducts with milk. Cancers originating from ducts are known as ductal carcinomas; those originating from lobules are known as lobular carcinomas.

Folk medicine	Folk medicine refers to healing practices and ideas of body physiology and health preservation widely known to much of the population in a culture, transmitted informally as general knowledge, and practiced or applied by anyone in the culture . All cultures and societies have knowledge best described as Folk medicine. Folk medicine often coexists with formalized, education-based, and institutionalized systems of healing such as Western medicine or systems of traditional medicine like Ayurvedic and Chinese medicine, but is distinguishable from formalized or institutionalized healing systems.
Therapeutic touch	Therapeutic touch (commonly shortened to),) or Distance Healing, is an energy therapy claimed to promote healing and reduce pain and anxiety. Practitioners of Therapeutic touch claim that by placing their hands on, or near, a patient, they are able to detect and manipulate the patient's putative energy field. Although there are currently (September 2009) 259 articles concerning Therapeutic touch on PubMed the quality of controlled research and tests is variable.
Cardiovascular disease	Cardiovascular disease or Cardiovascular diseases refers to the class of diseases that involve the heart or blood vessels (arteries and veins). While the term technically refers to any disease that affects the cardiovascular system (as used in MeSH), it is usually used to refer to those related to atherosclerosis (arterial disease). These conditions have similar causes, mechanisms, and treatments.
Health insurance	Health insurance is insurance that pays for medical expenses. It is sometimes used more broadly to include insurance covering disability or long-term nursing or custodial care needs. It may be provided through a government-sponsored social insurance program, or from private insurance companies.
Population health	Population health has been defined as 'the health outcomes of a group of individuals, including the distribution of such outcomes within the group.' It is an approach to health that aims to improve the health of an entire population. One major step in achieving this aim is to reduce health inequities among population groups. Population health seeks to step beyond the individual-level focus of mainstream medicine and public health by addressing a broad range of factors that impact health on a population-level, such as environment, social structure, resource distribution, etc.
Lead poisoning	Lead poisoning is a medical condition caused by increased levels of the heavy metal lead in the body. Lead interferes with a variety of body processes and is toxic to many organs and tissues including the heart, bones, intestines, kidneys, and reproductive and nervous systems. It interferes with the development of the nervous system and is therefore particularly toxic to children, causing potentially permanent learning and behavior disorders.
Maternal death	Maternal death also 'obstetrical death' is the death of a woman during or shortly after a pregnancy.

Chapter 2. Emerging Populations and Health,

	In 2000, the United Nations estimated global maternal mortality at 529,000, of which less than 1% occurred in the developed world. However, most of these deaths have been medically preventable for decades, because treatments to avoid such deaths have been well known since the 1950s.
Prenatal care	Prenatal care refers to the medical and nursing care recommended for women before and during pregnancy. The aim of good Prenatal care is to detect any potential problems early, to prevent them if possible (through recommendations on adequate nutrition, exercise, vitamin intake etc), and to direct the woman to appropriate specialists, hospitals, etc. if necessary.
Blood pressure	Blood pressure is the pressure (force per unit area) exerted by circulating blood on the walls of blood vessels, and constitutes one of the principal vital signs. The pressure of the circulating blood decreases as it moves away from the heart through arteries and capillaries, and toward the heart through veins. When unqualified, the term Blood pressure usually refers to brachial arterial pressure: that is, in the major blood vessel of the upper left or right arm that takes blood away from the heart.
Alcohol abuse	Alcohol abuse, as described in the DSM-IV, is a psychiatric diagnosis describing the recurring use of alcoholic beverages despite negative consequences. It is differentiated from alcohol dependence by the lack of symptoms such as tolerance and withdrawal. Alcohol abuse is sometimes referred to by the less specific term alcoholism.
Medicine Man	'Medicine Man' or 'Medicine woman' are English terms used to describe Native American healers and spiritual figures. Anthropologists tend to prefer the term 'shaman.'
	The primary function of these 'medicine elders' is to secure the help of the spirit world, including the Great Spirit (Wakan Tanka in the language of the Lakota Sioux), for the benefit of the entire community.
	Sometimes the help sought may be for the sake of healing disease, sometimes it may be for the sake of healing the psyche, sometimes the goal is to promote harmony between human groups or between humans & nature.
Case study	A Case study is a research methodology common in social science. It is based on an in-depth investigation of a single individual, group, or event to explore causation in order to find underlying principles.
Community health	Community health, a field within public health, is a discipline that concerns itself with the study and betterment of the health characteristics of biological communities. While the term community can be broadly defined, Community health tends to focus on geographic areas rather than people with shared characteristics.

| Ambulatory care | Ambulatory care is any medical care delivered on an outpatient basis. Many medical conditions do not require hospital admission and can be managed without admission to a hospital. Many medical investigations can be performed on an ambulatory basis, including blood tests, X-rays, endoscopy and even biopsy procedures of superficial organs. |

CHAPTER QUIZ: KEY TERMS, PEOPLE, PLACES, CONCEPTS

1. _____ refers to a range of pragmatic and evidence-based public health policies designed to reduce the harmful consequences associated with drug use and other high risk activities .

   Many advocates argue that prohibitionist laws criminalize people for suffering from a disease and cause harm, for example by obliging drug addicts to obtain drugs of unknown purity from unreliable criminal sources at high prices, increasing the risk of overdose and death. .

   a. Wernicke-Korsakoff syndrome
   b. Bacteriophage
   c. Harm reduction
   d. Benign prostatic hyperplasia

2. _____ is the profession of educating people about health. Areas within this profession encompass environmental health, physical health, social health, emotional health, intellectual health, and spiritual health. It can be defined as the principle by which individuals and groups of people learn to behave in a manner conducive to the promotion, maintenance, or restoration of health.

   a. Mahatma Gandhi Institute of Medical Sciences
   b. Centers for Public Health Preparedness
   c. Health education
   d. Mark Lester

3. _____ is a measure of the number of deaths (in general,) in some population, scaled to the size of that population, per unit time. _____ is typically expressed in units of deaths per 1000 individuals per year; thus, a _____ of 9.5 in a population of 100,000 would mean 950 deaths per year in that entire population. It is distinct from morbidity rate, which refers to the number of individuals in poor health during a given time period (the prevalence rate) or the number who currently have that disease (the incidence rate), scaled to the size of the population.

   a. Mortality rate
   b. Centers for Public Health Preparedness
   c. Baroreflex
   d. Benign prostatic hyperplasia

Visit Cram101.com for full Practice Exams

Chapter 2. Emerging Populations and Health,

4. _____, a field within public health, is a discipline that concerns itself with the study and betterment of the health characteristics of biological communities. While the term community can be broadly defined, _____ tends to focus on geographic areas rather than people with shared characteristics. The health characteristics of a community are often examined using geographic information system (GIS) software and public health datasets.

    a. Bacteriophage
    b. Alcohol dependence
    c. Community health
    d. Alcoholic liver disease

5. _____, or potty training, is the process of training a young child to use the toilet for urination and defecation, though training may start with a smaller toilet bowl-shaped device (often known as a potty). In Western countries it is usually started and completed between the ages of 12 months and three years with boys typically being at the higher end of the age spectrum.

Cultural factors play a large part in what age is deemed appropriate, with the age being generally later in America.

Most advise that _____ is a mutual task, requiring cooperation, agreement and understanding between child and the caregiver, and the best potty training techniques emphasize consistency and positive reinforcement over punishment - making it fun for the child.

    a. Bacteriophage
    b. Centers for Public Health Preparedness
    c. Baroreflex
    d. Toilet training

1. c
2. c
3. a
4. c
5. d

You can take the complete Chapter Practice Test

for Chapter 2. Emerging Populations and Health,
on all key terms, persons, places, and concepts.

Online 99 Cents

http://www.epub1625.32.20273.2.cram101.com/

Use www.Cram101.com for all your study needs

including Cram101's online interactive problem solving labs in

chemistry, statistics, mathematics, and more.

Chapter 3. Health Policy and the Delivery System,

CHAPTER OUTLINE: KEY TERMS, PEOPLE, PLACES, CONCEPTS

Health care

Health insurance

Mortality rate

National health insurance

Population health

Case study

Life expectancy

Institute of Medicine

Florence Nightingale

Public health

Infectious disease

Louis Pasteur

Staphylococcus aureus

Health disparities

Cultural competence

Fee-for-service

Primary care

Health maintenance organization

Independent practice association

_____ | Managed care

_____ | Point of service plan

_____ | Preferred Provider Organization

_____ | Disease registry

_____ | Food and Drug Administration

_____ | Mental health

_____ | Substance abuse

_____ | Medical savings account

_____ | Health system

_____ | Home birth

_____ | Nursing home

_____ | Prescription drug

_____ | Home care

_____ | Temporary Assistance for Needy Families

Health care	Health care , refers to the treatment and management of illness, and the preservation of health through services offered by the medical, dental, complementary and alternative medicine, pharmaceutical, clinical laboratory sciences , nursing, and allied health professions. Health care embraces all the goods and services designed to promote health, including 'preventive, curative and palliative interventions, whether directed to individuals or to populations'.
	Before the term Health care became popular, English-speakers referred to medicine or to the health sector and spoke of the treatment and prevention of illness and disease.
Health insurance	Health insurance is insurance that pays for medical expenses. It is sometimes used more broadly to include insurance covering disability or long-term nursing or custodial care needs. It may be provided through a government-sponsored social insurance program, or from private insurance companies.
Mortality rate	Mortality rate is a measure of the number of deaths (in general,) in some population, scaled to the size of that population, per unit time. Mortality rate is typically expressed in units of deaths per 1000 individuals per year; thus, a Mortality rate of 9.5 in a population of 100,000 would mean 950 deaths per year in that entire population. It is distinct from morbidity rate, which refers to the number of individuals in poor health during a given time period (the prevalence rate) or the number who currently have that disease (the incidence rate), scaled to the size of the population.
National health insurance	National health insurance is health insurance that insures a national population for the costs of health care and usually is instituted as a program of healthcare reform. It may be administered by the public sector, the private sector, or a combination of both. Funding mechanisms vary with the particular program and country.
Population health	Population health has been defined as 'the health outcomes of a group of individuals, including the distribution of such outcomes within the group.' It is an approach to health that aims to improve the health of an entire population. One major step in achieving this aim is to reduce health inequities among population groups. Population health seeks to step beyond the individual-level focus of mainstream medicine and public health by addressing a broad range of factors that impact health on a population-level, such as environment, social structure, resource distribution, etc.
Case study	A Case study is a research methodology common in social science. It is based on an in-depth investigation of a single individual, group, or event to explore causation in order to find underlying principles.
Life expectancy	Life expectancy is the average number of years of life remaining at a given age. The term is most often used in the human context, but used also in plant or animal ecology and the calculation is based on the analysis of life tables (also known as actuarial tables).

Chapter 3. Health Policy and the Delivery System,

Institute of Medicine	The Institute of Medicine, one of the United States National Academies, is a not-for-profit, non-governmental American organization chartered in 1970 as a part of the United States National Academy of Sciences. Its purpose is to provide national advice on issues relating to biomedical science, medicine, and health, and its mission to serve as adviser to the nation to improve health. It works outside the framework of the U.S. federal government to provide independent guidance and analysis and relies on a volunteer workforce of scientists and other experts, operating under a rigorous, formal peer-review system.
Florence Nightingale	Florence Nightingale, OM, RRC was an English nurse, writer and statistician. She came to prominence during the Crimean War for her pioneering work in nursing, and was dubbed 'The Lady with the Lamp' after her habit of making rounds at night to tend injured soldiers. Nightingale laid the foundation of professional nursing with the establishment, in 1860, of her nursing school at St Thomas's Hospital in London, the first secular nursing school in the world.
Public health	Public health is 'the science and art of preventing disease, prolonging life and promoting health through the organized efforts and informed choices of society, organizations, public and private, communities and individuals.' (1920, C.E.A. Winslow) It is concerned with threats to the overall health of a community based on population health analysis. The population in question can be as small as a handful of people or as large as all the inhabitants of several continents (for instance, in the case of a pandemic). Public health is typically divided into epidemiology, biostatistics and health services.
Infectious disease	Infectious diseases, also known as communicable diseases, or transmissible diseases comprise clinically evident illness (i.e., characteristic medical signs and/or symptoms of disease) resulting from the infection, presence and growth of pathogenic biological agents in an individual host organism. In certain cases, infectious diseases may be asymtomatic for much or all of their course. Infectious pathogens include some viruses, bacteria, fungi, protozoa, multicellular parasites, and aberrant proteins known as prions.
Louis Pasteur	Louis Pasteur was a French chemist and microbiologist born in Dole. He is best known for his remarkable breakthroughs in the causes and preventions of disease. His discoveries reduced mortality from puerperal fever, and he created the first vaccine for rabies.
Staphylococcus aureus	Staphylococcus aureus is a facultatively anaerobic, gram positive coccus and is the most common cause of staph infections. It is a spherical bacterium, frequently part of the skin flora found in the nose and on skin. About 20% of the population are long-term carriers of S. aureus.
Health disparities	Health disparities refer to gaps in the quality of health and health care across racial, ethnic, sexual orientation and socioeconomic groups. The Health Resources and Services Administration defines Health disparities as 'population-specific differences in the presence of disease, health outcomes, or access to health care.'

	In the United States, Health disparities are well documented in minority populations such as African Americans, Native Americans, Asian Americans, and Latinos. When compared to whites, these minority groups have higher incidence of chronic diseases, higher mortality, and poorer health outcomes.
Cultural competence	Cultural competence refers to an ability to interact effectively with people of different cultures. Cultural competence comprises four components: (a) Awareness of one's own cultural worldview, (b) Attitude towards cultural differences, (c) Knowledge of different cultural practices and worldviews, and (d) cross-cultural skills. Developing Cultural competence results in an ability to understand, communicate with, and effectively interact with people across cultures.
Fee-for-service	Fee-for-service is a standard business model where services are unbundled and paid for separately. In the health insurance and the health care industries, Fee-for-service occurs when doctors and other health care providers receive a fee for each service such as an office visit, test, procedure, or other health care service. Fee-for-service health insurance plans typically allow patients to obtain care from doctors or hospitals of their choosing, but in return for this flexibility they may pay higher copayments or deductibles.
Primary care	Primary care is a term used for the activity of a health care provider who acts as a first point of consultation for all patients. Continuity of care is also a key characteristic of Primary care. Primary care is an important form of health access for patients.
Health maintenance organization	A Health maintenance organization is a type of managed care organization (MCO) that provides a form of health care coverage in the United States that is fulfilled through hospitals, doctors, and other providers with which the Health maintenance organization has a contract. The Health maintenance organization Act of 1973 required employers with 25 or more employees to offer federally certified Health maintenance organization options. Unlike traditional indemnity insurance, an Health maintenance organization covers only care rendered by those doctors and other professionals who have agreed to treat patients in accordance with the Health maintenance organization's guidelines and restrictions in exchange for a steady stream of customers.
Independent practice association	An Independent practice association is an association of independent physicians, or other organization that contracts with independent physicians, and provides services to managed care organizations on a negotiated per capita rate, flat retainer fee, or negotiated fee-for-service basis.

Chapter 3. Health Policy and the Delivery System,

An HMO or other managed care plan may contract with an Independent practice association which in turn contracts with independent physicians to treat members at discounted fees or on a capitation basis. The typical Independent practice association encompasses all specialties, but an Independent practice association can be solely for primary care or may be single specialty.

Managed care

The term Managed care is used to describe a variety of techniques intended to reduce the cost of providing health benefits and improve the quality of care ('Managed care techniques') f), or to describe systems of financing and delivering health care to enrollees organized around Managed care techniques and concepts ('Managed care delivery systems'). According to the United States National Library of Medicine, the term 'Managed care' encompasses programs: '

...intended to reduce unnecessary health care costs through a variety of mechanisms, including: economic incentives for physicians and patients to select less costly forms of care; programs for reviewing the medical necessity of specific services; increased beneficiary cost sharing; controls on inpatient admissions and lengths of stay; the establishment of cost-sharing incentives for outpatient surgery; selective contracting with health care providers; and the intensive management of high-cost health care cases. The programs may be provided in a variety of settings, such as Health Maintenance Organizations and Preferred Provider Organizations.

Point of service plan

A Point of service plan is a type of managed care health insurance system. It combines characteristics of both the HMO and the PPO. Members of a POS plan do not make a choice about which system to use until the point at which the service is being used. .

Preferred Provider Organization

In health insurance in the United States, a Preferred Provider Organization is a managed care organization of medical doctors, hospitals, and other health care providers who have covenanted with an insurer or a third-party administrator to provide health care at reduced rates to the insurer's or administrator's clients.

A Preferred Provider Organization is a subscription-based medical care arrangement. A membership allows a substantial discount below their regularly charged rates from the designated professionals partnered with the organization.

Disease registry

Disease registries are databases that collect clinical data on patients with a specific disease (diabetes, asthma, CHF, hypertension, etc) or keep track of specific medical tests (pap smear, mammogram).

In its most simple form, a Disease registry could consist of a collection of paper cards kept inside 'a shoe box' by a individual physician.

Food and Drug Administration	The Food and Drug Administration is an agency of the United States Department of Health and Human Services, one of the United States federal executive departments, responsible for protecting and promoting public health through the regulation and supervision of food safety, tobacco products, dietary supplements, prescription and over-the-counter pharmaceutical drugs (medications), vaccines, biopharmaceuticals, blood transfusions, medical devices, electromagnetic radiation emitting devices (ERED), veterinary products, and cosmetics. The FDA also enforces other laws, notably Section 361 of the Public Health Service Act and associated regulations, many of which are not directly related to food or drugs. These include sanitation requirements on interstate travel and control of disease on products ranging from certain household pets to sperm donation for assisted reproduction.
Mental health	Mental health is a term used to describe either a level of cognitive or emotional well-being or an absence of a mental disorder. From perspectives of the discipline of positive psychology or holism Mental health may include an individual's ability to enjoy life and procure a balance between life activities and efforts to achieve psychological resilience. The World Health Organization defines Mental health as 'a state of well-being in which the individual realizes his or her own abilities, can cope with the normal stresses of life, can work productively and fruitfully, and is able to make a contribution to his or her community'.
Substance abuse	Substance abuse also known as drug abuse, refers to a maladaptive pattern of use of a substance that is not considered dependent. The term 'drug abuse' does not exclude dependency, but is otherwise used in a similar manner in nonmedical contexts. The terms have a huge range of definitions related to taking a psychoactive drug or performance enhancing drug for a non-therapeutic or non-medical effect.
Medical savings account	Medical savings account refers to an account in which tax-deferred deposits can be made for medical expenses. Medisave was introduced in April 1984 as a national medical savings system for Singaporeans. The system allows Singaporeans to put aside part of their income into a Medisave account to meet future personal or immediate family's hospitalization, day surgery and for certain outpatient expenses.
Health system	A Health System can be defined as the structured and interrelated set of all actors and institutions contributing to health improvement. The health system boundaries could then be referred to the concept of health action, which is 'any set of activities whose primary intent is to improve or maintain health' . A wide concept

Chapter 3. Health Policy and the Delivery System,

Home birth	A Home birth is a birth that is planned to occur at home. It is contrasted to birth that occur in a hospital or a birth centre. Homebirths are divided into two types -- attended and unattended births.
Nursing home	A Nursing home, convalescent home, Skilled Nursing Unit (SNU), care home or rest home provides a type of care of residents: it is a place of residence for people who require constant nursing care and have significant deficiencies with activities of daily living. Residents include the elderly and younger adults with physical or mental disabilities. Eligible adults 18 or older can stay in a skilled nursing facility to receive physical, occupational, and other rehabilitative therapies following an accident or illness.
Prescription drug	A Prescription drug is a licensed medicine that is regulated by legislation to require a prescription before it can be obtained. The term is used to distinguish it from over-the-counter drugs which can be obtained without a prescription. Different jurisdictions have different definitions of what constitutes a Prescription drug.
Home care	Home care, (commonly referred to as domiciliary care), is health care , it is also known as skilled care) or by family and friends (also known as caregivers, primary caregiver, or voluntary caregivers who give informal care). Often, the term Home care is used to distinguish non-medical care or custodial care, which is care that is provided by persons who are not nurses, doctors, or other licensed medical personnel, whereas the term home health care, refers to care that is provided by licensed personnel. 'Home care', 'home health care', 'in-Home care' are phrases that are used interchangeably in the United States to mean any type of care given to a person in their own home.
Temporary Assistance for Needy Families	Temporary Assistance for Needy Families is one of the United States of America's federal assistance programs. It began on July 1, 1997, and succeeded the Aid to Families with Dependent Children (AFDC) program, providing cash assistance to indigent American families with dependent children through the United States Department of Health and Human Services. Prior to 1997, the federal government designed the overall program requirements and guidelines, while states administered the program and determined eligibility for benefits.

1. _____ is the average number of years of life remaining at a given age. The term is most often used in the human context, but used also in plant or animal ecology and the calculation is based on the analysis of life tables (also known as actuarial tables). The term may also be used in the context of manufactured objects although the related term shelf life is used for consumer products and the term mean time to breakdown (MTTB) is used in engineering literature.

   a. Maximum life span
   b. Life expectancy
   c. Mark Lester
   d. Self-funded health care

2. _____ is a measure of the number of deaths (in general,) in some population, scaled to the size of that population, per unit time. _____ is typically expressed in units of deaths per 1000 individuals per year; thus, a _____ of 9.5 in a population of 100,000 would mean 950 deaths per year in that entire population. It is distinct from morbidity rate, which refers to the number of individuals in poor health during a given time period (the prevalence rate) or the number who currently have that disease (the incidence rate), scaled to the size of the population.

   a. Mortality rate
   b. Baroreflex
   c. Benign prostatic hyperplasia
   d. Benzathine benzylpenicillin

3. _____ , refers to the treatment and management of illness, and the preservation of health through services offered by the medical, dental, complementary and alternative medicine, pharmaceutical, clinical laboratory sciences , nursing, and allied health professions. _____ embraces all the goods and services designed to promote health, including 'preventive, curative and palliative interventions, whether directed to individuals or to populations'.

   Before the term _____ became popular, English-speakers referred to medicine or to the health sector and spoke of the treatment and prevention of illness and disease.

   a. Bacteriophage
   b. Baroreflex
   c. Health care
   d. Benzathine benzylpenicillin

4. _____ is insurance that pays for medical expenses. It is sometimes used more broadly to include insurance covering disability or long-term nursing or custodial care needs. It may be provided through a government-sponsored social insurance program, or from private insurance companies.

   a. Bacteriophage
   b. Health insurance
   c. Benign prostatic hyperplasia
   d. Benzathine benzylpenicillin

5. . _____ has been defined as 'the health outcomes of a group of individuals, including the distribution of such outcomes within the group.' It is an approach to health that aims to improve the health of an entire population.

One major step in achieving this aim is to reduce health inequities among population groups. _____ seeks to step beyond the individual-level focus of mainstream medicine and public health by addressing a broad range of factors that impact health on a population-level, such as environment, social structure, resource distribution, etc.

a. Public health insurance option
b. Roemer's law
c. Population health
d. Self-funded health care

1. b
2. a
3. c
4. b
5. c

You can take the complete Chapter Practice Test

for Chapter 3. Health Policy and the Delivery System,
on all key terms, persons, places, and concepts.

Online 99 Cents

http://www.epub1625.32.20273.3.cram101.com/

Use www.Cram101.com for all your study needs

including Cram101's online interactive problem solving labs in

chemistry, statistics, mathematics, and more.

Chapter 4. The Therapeutic Relationship,

CHAPTER OUTLINE: KEY TERMS, PEOPLE, PLACES, CONCEPTS

	Therapeutic relationship
	Health promotion
	Therapeutic touch
	Telehealth
	Communication
	Personal space
	Health care
	Health effect
	Obstacle
	Health literacy

CHAPTER HIGHLIGHTS & NOTES: KEY TERMS, PEOPLE, PLACES, CONCEPTS

Therapeutic relationship	The Therapeutic relationship the therapeutic alliance, and the working alliance, refers to the relationship between a mental health professional and a patient. It is the means by which the professional hopes to engage with, and effect change in, a patient. While much early work on this subject was generated from a psychodynamic perspective, researchers from other orientations have since investigated this area.
Health promotion	Health promotion has been defined by the World Health Organization's 2005 Bangkok Charter for Health promotion in a Globalized World as 'the process of enabling people to increase control over their health and its determinants, and thereby improve their health'.

Visit Cram101.com for full Practice Exams

	The primary means of Health promotion occur through developing healthy public policy that addresses the prerequisites of health such as income, housing, food security, employment, and quality working conditions. There is a tendency among public health officials and governments -- and this is especially the case in liberal nations such as Canada and the USA -- to reduce Health promotion to health education and social marketing focused on changing behavioral risk factors.
Therapeutic touch	Therapeutic touch (commonly shortened to),) or Distance Healing, is an energy therapy claimed to promote healing and reduce pain and anxiety. Practitioners of Therapeutic touch claim that by placing their hands on, or near, a patient, they are able to detect and manipulate the patient's putative energy field. Although there are currently (September 2009) 259 articles concerning Therapeutic touch on PubMed the quality of controlled research and tests is variable.
Telehealth	Telehealth is the delivery of health-related services and information via telecommunications technologies. Telehealth delivery could be as simple as two health professionals discussing a case over the telephone, or as sophisticated as using videoconferencing between providers at facilities in two countries, or even as complex as robotic technology. Telehealth is an expansion of telemedicine, and unlike telemedicine (which more narrowly focuses on the curative aspect) it encompasses preventive, promotive and curative aspects.
Communication	Communication is a process of transferring information from one entity to another. Communication processes are sign-mediated interactions between at least two agents which share a repertoire of signs and semiotic rules. Communication is commonly defined as 'the imparting or interchange of thoughts, opinions, or information by speech, writing, or signs'.
Personal space	Personal space is the region surrounding a person which they regard as psychologically theirs. Invasion of Personal space often leads to discomfort, anger, or anxiety on the part of the victim. The notion of Personal space comes from Edward T. Hall, whose ideas were influenced by Heini Hediger's studies of behavior of zoo animals.
Health care	Health care , refers to the treatment and management of illness, and the preservation of health through services offered by the medical, dental, complementary and alternative medicine, pharmaceutical, clinical laboratory sciences , nursing, and allied health professions. Health care embraces all the goods and services designed to promote health, including 'preventive, curative and palliative interventions, whether directed to individuals or to populations'. Before the term Health care became popular, English-speakers referred to medicine or to the health sector and spoke of the treatment and prevention of illness and disease.
Health effect	Health effects are changes in health resulting from exposure to a source.

Health effects are an important consideration in many areas, such as hygiene, pollution studies, workplace safety, nutrition and health sciences in general. Some of the major environmental sources of Health effects are air pollution, water pollution, soil contamination, noise pollution and over-illumination.

Obstacle	An obstacle, is an object, thing, action or situation that causes an obstruction, forms a barrier, creates a difficulty, a nuisance or a disorder to achieve concrete goals. There are, therefore, different types of obstacles, which can be physical, economic, biopsychosocial, cultural, political, technological or even military. Physical barriers As physical obstacles, we can enumerate all those physical barriers that block the action and prevent the progress or the achievement of a concrete goal.
Health literacy	Health literacy is an individual's ability to read, understand and use healthcare information to make decisions and follow instructions for treatment. There are multiple definitions of Health literacy, in part because Health literacy involves both the context (or setting) in which Health literacy demands are made (e.g., health care, media, Internet or fitness facility) and the skills that people bring to that situation (Rudd, Moeykens, & Colton, 1999). Studies reveal that up to half of patients cannot understand basic healthcare information.

1. _____ is the delivery of health-related services and information via telecommunications technologies. _____ delivery could be as simple as two health professionals discussing a case over the telephone, or as sophisticated as using videoconferencing between providers at facilities in two countries, or even as complex as robotic technology.

   _____ is an expansion of telemedicine, and unlike telemedicine (which more narrowly focuses on the curative aspect) it encompasses preventive, promotive and curative aspects.

   a. Telephone interpreting
   b. Telepresence
   c. Telehealth
   d. Text over IP

2. . The _____ the therapeutic alliance, and the working alliance, refers to the relationship between a mental health professional and a patient. It is the means by which the professional hopes to engage with, and effect change in, a patient.

While much early work on this subject was generated from a psychodynamic perspective, researchers from other orientations have since investigated this area.

a. Peer support
b. Bacteriophage
c. Baroreflex
d. Therapeutic relationship

3. _____ , refers to the treatment and management of illness, and the preservation of health through services offered by the medical, dental, complementary and alternative medicine, pharmaceutical, clinical laboratory sciences , nursing, and allied health professions. _____ embraces all the goods and services designed to promote health, including 'preventive, curative and palliative interventions, whether directed to individuals or to populations'.

Before the term _____ became popular, English-speakers referred to medicine or to the health sector and spoke of the treatment and prevention of illness and disease.

a. Bacteriophage
b. Baroreflex
c. Health care
d. Text over IP

4. _____ has been defined by the World Health Organization's 2005 Bangkok Charter for _____ in a Globalized World as 'the process of enabling people to increase control over their health and its determinants, and thereby improve their health'. The primary means of _____ occur through developing healthy public policy that addresses the prerequisities of health such as income, housing, food security, employment, and quality working conditions. There is a tendency among public health officials and governments -- and this is especially the case in liberal nations such as Canada and the USA -- to reduce _____ to health education and social marketing focused on changing behavioral risk factors.

a. Bacteriophage
b. Baroreflex
c. Health promotion
d. Benzathine benzylpenicillin

5. _____ is a process of transferring information from one entity to another. _____ processes are sign-mediated interactions between at least two agents which share a repertoire of signs and semiotic rules. _____ is commonly defined as 'the imparting or interchange of thoughts, opinions, or information by speech, writing, or signs'.

a. Sleepwalking
b. Bacteriophage
c. Baroreflex
d. Communication

1. c
2. d
3. c
4. c
5. d

You can take the complete Chapter Practice Test

for Chapter 4. The Therapeutic Relationship,
on all key terms, persons, places, and concepts.

Online 99 Cents

http://www.epub1625.32.20273.4.cram101.com/

Use www.Cram101.com for all your study needs

including Cram101's online interactive problem solving labs in

chemistry, statistics, mathematics, and more.

CHAPTER OUTLINE: KEY TERMS, PEOPLE, PLACES, CONCEPTS

_____ Health promotion

_____ Health care

_____ Genetic counseling

_____ Cardiovascular disease

_____ Obstacle

_____ Advocacy

_____ Problem solving

_____ Health care proxy

_____ Informed consent

_____ Health system

_____ Health insurance

_____ Terminal illness

_____ Transtheoretical model

_____ Social justice

_____ Examination

_____ Case study

_____ Chronic pain

_____ Depression

Chapter 5. Ethical Issues Relevant to Health Promotion,

Health promotion	Health promotion has been defined by the World Health Organization's 2005 Bangkok Charter for Health promotion in a Globalized World as 'the process of enabling people to increase control over their health and its determinants, and thereby improve their health'. The primary means of Health promotion occur through developing healthy public policy that addresses the prerequisities of health such as income, housing, food security, employment, and quality working conditions. There is a tendency among public health officials and governments -- and this is especially the case in liberal nations such as Canada and the USA -- to reduce Health promotion to health education and social marketing focused on changing behavioral risk factors.
Health care	Health care , refers to the treatment and management of illness, and the preservation of health through services offered by the medical, dental, complementary and alternative medicine, pharmaceutical, clinical laboratory sciences , nursing, and allied health professions. Health care embraces all the goods and services designed to promote health, including 'preventive, curative and palliative interventions, whether directed to individuals or to populations'.
	Before the term Health care became popular, English-speakers referred to medicine or to the health sector and spoke of the treatment and prevention of illness and disease.
Genetic counseling	Genetic counseling is the process by which patients or relatives, at risk of an inherited disorder, are advised of the consequences and nature of the disorder, the probability of developing or transmitting it, and the options open to them in management and family planning in order to prevent, avoid or ameliorate it. This complex process can be seen from diagnostic (the actual estimation of risk) and supportive aspects.
	A genetic counselor is a medical genetics expert with a master of science degree.
Cardiovascular disease	Cardiovascular disease or Cardiovascular diseases refers to the class of diseases that involve the heart or blood vessels (arteries and veins). While the term technically refers to any disease that affects the cardiovascular system (as used in MeSH), it is usually used to refer to those related to atherosclerosis (arterial disease). These conditions have similar causes, mechanisms, and treatments.
Obstacle	An obstacle, is an object, thing, action or situation that causes an obstruction, forms a barrier, creates a difficulty, a nuisance or a disorder to achieve concrete goals. There are, therefore, different types of obstacles, which can be physical, economic, biopsychosocial, cultural, political, technological or even military.
	Physical barriers

Advocacy	Advocacy by an individual or by an Advocacy group normally aim to influence public-policy and resource allocation decisions within political, economic, and social systems and institutions; it may be motivated from moral, ethical or faith principles or simply to protect an asset of interest. Advocacy can include many activities that a person or organization undertakes including media campaigns, public speaking, commissioning and publishing research or poll or the 'filing of friend of the court briefs'. Lobbying (often by Lobby groups) is a form of Advocacy where a direct approach is made to legislators on an issue which plays a significant role in modern politics.
Problem solving	Problem solving is a mental process and is part of the larger problem process that includes problem finding and problem shaping. Considered the most complex of all intellectual functions, Problem solving has been defined as higher-order cognitive process that requires the modulation and control of more routine or fundamental skills. Problem solving occurs when an organism or an artificial intelligence system needs to move from a given state to a desired goal state.
Health care proxy	A Health care proxy is an instrument that allows a patient to appoint an agent to make health care decisions in the event that the primary individual is incapable of executing such decisions. Once the document is drafted, the primary individual continues to be allowed to make health care decisions as long as they are still competent to do so. Health care proxies are permitted in forty-nine states as well as the District of Columbia.
Informed consent	Informed consent is a legal condition whereby a person can be said to have given consent based upon a clear appreciation and understanding of the facts, implications and future consequences of an action. In order to give Informed consent, the individual concerned must have adequate reasoning faculties and be in possession of all relevant facts at the time consent is given. Impairments to reasoning and judgement which would make it impossible for someone to give Informed consent include such factors as severe mental retardation, severe mental illness, intoxication, severe sleep deprivation, Alzheimer's disease, or being in a coma.
Health system	A Health System can be defined as the structured and interrelated set of all actors and institutions contributing to health improvement. The health system boundaries could then be referred to the concept of health action, which is 'any set of activities whose primary intent is to improve or maintain health'. A wide concept Too often health systems have been defined with a reductionist perspective, for example reducing it to the health care systems.
Health insurance	Health insurance is insurance that pays for medical expenses. It is sometimes used more broadly to include insurance covering disability or long-term nursing or custodial care needs.

Chapter 5. Ethical Issues Relevant to Health Promotion,

Terminal illness	Terminal illness is a medical term popularized in the 20th century to describe an active and malignant disease that cannot be cured or adequately treated and that is reasonably expected to result in the death of the patient. This term is more commonly used for progressive diseases such as cancer or advanced heart disease than for trauma. In popular use, it indicates a disease which will end the life of the sufferer.
Transtheoretical model	The Transtheoretical model in health psychology is intended to explain or predict a person's success or failure in achieving a proposed behavior change, such as developing different habits. It attempts to answer why the change 'stuck' or alternatively why the change was not made. The Transtheoretical model is also known by the acronym 'TTranstheoretical model' and by the term 'stages of change model'.
Social justice	Social justice is the application of the concept of justice on a social scale. The term 'Social justice' was coined by the Jesuit Luigi Taparelli in the 1840s. The idea was elaborated by the moral theologian John A. Ryan, who initiated the concept of a living wage.
Examination	A competitive Examination is an Examination where applicants compete for a limited number of positions, as opposed to merely having to reach a certain level to pass. A comprehensive Examination is a specific type of exam taken by graduate students, which may determine their eligibility to continue their studies. In the UK an Examination is usually supervised by an invigilator.
Case study	A Case study is a research methodology common in social science. It is based on an in-depth investigation of a single individual, group, or event to explore causation in order to find underlying principles.
Chronic pain	Chronic pain is defined as pain that persists longer than the temporal course of natural healing, associated with a particular type of injury or disease process. The International Association for the Study of Pain defines pain as 'an unpleasant sensory and emotional experience associated with actual or potential tissue damage, or described in terms of such damage.' Pain is subjective in nature and is defined by the person experiencing it, and the medical community's understanding of Chronic pain now includes the impact that the mind has in processing and interpreting pain signals.

Depression	Depression is a state of low mood and aversion to activity that can affect a person's thoughts, behaviour, feelings and physical well-being. It may include feelings of sadness, anxiety, emptiness, hopelessness, worthlessness, guilt, irritability, or restlessness. Depressed people may lose interest in activities that once were pleasurable, experience difficulty concentrating, remembering details, or making decisions, and may contemplate or attempt suicide.

CHAPTER QUIZ: KEY TERMS, PEOPLE, PLACES, CONCEPTS

1. _____ is the application of the concept of justice on a social scale.

   The term '_____' was coined by the Jesuit Luigi Taparelli in the 1840s. The idea was elaborated by the moral theologian John A. Ryan, who initiated the concept of a living wage.

   a. Bacteriophage
   b. Deinstitutionalisation
   c. Chiroplasty
   d. Social justice

2. _____ is a legal condition whereby a person can be said to have given consent based upon a clear appreciation and understanding of the facts, implications and future consequences of an action. In order to give _____, the individual concerned must have adequate reasoning faculties and be in possession of all relevant facts at the time consent is given. Impairments to reasoning and judgement which would make it impossible for someone to give _____ include such factors as severe mental retardation, severe mental illness, intoxication, severe sleep deprivation, Alzheimer's disease, or being in a coma.

   a. Electronic Common Technical Document
   b. EUDRANET
   c. Informed consent
   d. EudraLex

3. _____ is a mental process and is part of the larger problem process that includes problem finding and problem shaping. Considered the most complex of all intellectual functions, _____ has been defined as higher-order cognitive process that requires the modulation and control of more routine or fundamental skills. _____ occurs when an organism or an artificial intelligence system needs to move from a given state to a desired goal state.

   a. Bacteriophage
   b. EUPHIX
   c. Problem solving
   d. Emperor's College

4. A competitive _____ is an _____ where applicants compete for a limited number of positions, as opposed to merely having to reach a certain level to pass.

   A comprehensive _____ is a specific type of exam taken by graduate students, which may determine their eligibility to continue their studies.

   In the UK an _____ is usually supervised by an invigilator.

   a. abdominal exam
   b. Deinstitutionalisation
   c. Chiroplasty
   d. Examination

5. _____ has been defined by the World Health Organization's 2005 Bangkok Charter for _____ in a Globalized World as 'the process of enabling people to increase control over their health and its determinants, and thereby improve their health'. The primary means of _____ occur through developing healthy public policy that addresses the prerequisities of health such as income, housing, food security, employment, and quality working conditions. There is a tendency among public health officials and governments -- and this is especially the case in liberal nations such as Canada and the USA -- to reduce _____ to health education and social marketing focused on changing behavioral risk factors.

   a. Bacteriophage
   b. Baroreflex
   c. Benign prostatic hyperplasia
   d. Health promotion

ANSWER KEY
Chapter 5. Ethical Issues Relevant to Health Promotion,

---

1. d
2. c
3. c
4. d
5. d

You can take the complete Chapter Practice Test

for Chapter 5. Ethical Issues Relevant to Health Promotion,
on all key terms, persons, places, and concepts.

Online 99 Cents

http://www.epub1625.32.20273.5.cram101.com/

Use www.Cram101.com for all your study needs

including Cram101's online interactive problem solving labs in

chemistry, statistics, mathematics, and more.

CHAPTER OUTLINE: KEY TERMS, PEOPLE, PLACES, CONCEPTS

_____ | Health promotion

_____ | Nursing diagnosis

_____ | Health care

_____ | Coma scale

_____ | Mini-mental state examination

_____ | Pain scale

_____ | Human development

_____ | Gender identity

_____ | Sex education

_____ | Data collection

_____ | Risk factor

_____ | Cardiovascular disease

CHAPTER HIGHLIGHTS & NOTES: KEY TERMS, PEOPLE, PLACES, CONCEPTS

Health promotion	Health promotion has been defined by the World Health Organization's 2005 Bangkok Charter for Health promotion in a Globalized World as 'the process of enabling people to increase control over their health and its determinants, and thereby improve their health'. The primary means of Health promotion occur through developing healthy public policy that addresses the prerequisites of health such as income, housing, food security, employment, and quality working conditions.

Chapter 6. Health Promotion and the Individual,

Nursing diagnosis	A Nursing diagnosis is a standardized statement about the health of a client (who can be an individual, a family, or a community) for the purpose of providing nursing care. Nursing diagnoses are developed based on data obtained during the nursing assessment. The main organization for defining standard diagnoses in North America is the North American Nursing diagnosis Association, now known as NANDA-International.
Health care	Health care , refers to the treatment and management of illness, and the preservation of health through services offered by the medical, dental, complementary and alternative medicine, pharmaceutical, clinical laboratory sciences , nursing, and allied health professions. Health care embraces all the goods and services designed to promote health, including 'preventive, curative and palliative interventions, whether directed to individuals or to populations'. Before the term Health care became popular, English-speakers referred to medicine or to the health sector and spoke of the treatment and prevention of illness and disease.
Coma scale	A Coma scale is a system to assess the severity of coma. There are several such systems: The Glasgow Coma scale is neurological scale which aims to give a reliable, objective way of recording the conscious state of a person, for initial as well as continuing assessment. A patient is assessed against the criteria of the scale, and the resulting points give a patient score between 3 (indicating deep unconsciousness) and either 14 (original scale) or 15 (the more widely used modified or revised scale).
Mini-mental state examination	The Mini-mental state examination (MMini-mental state examination) or Folstein test is a brief 30-point questionnaire test that is used to screen for cognitive impairment. It is commonly used in medicine to screen for dementia. It is also used to estimate the severity of cognitive impairment at a given point in time and to follow the course of cognitive changes in an individual over time, thus making it an effective way to document an individual's response to treatment.
Pain scale	A pain scale measures a patient's pain intensity or other features. Pain scales are based on self-report, observational (behavioral), or physiological data. Self-report is considered primary and should be obtained if possible.
Human development	Human development is the process of growing to maturity. In biological terms, this entails growth from a one-celled zygote to an adult human being.

Gender identity	Gender identity refers to one's chosen social identity from amongst the acknowledged gender identities present in a society, that to represent one's sex and gender aspirations. A person's Gender identity is the combination of one's outer sex, as represented by one's genitalia, and one's inner sex, i.e. the inner sense of being a male or a female.
	One's inner sex is also referred to as 'Gender' (as distinct from 'sex' which refers to one's outer sex).
Sex education	Sex education is a broad term used to describe education about human sexual anatomy, sexual reproduction, sexual intercourse, reproductive health, emotional relations, reproductive rights and responsibilities, abstinence, contraception, and other aspects of human sexual behavior. Common avenues for sex education are parents or caregivers, school programs, and public health campaigns.
	Overview
	Sex education may also be described as 'sexuality education', which means that it encompasses education about all aspects of sexuality, including information about family planning, reproduction (fertilization, conception and development of the embryo and fetus, through to childbirth), plus information about all aspects of one's sexuality including: body image, sexual orientation, sexual pleasure, values, decision making, communication, dating, relationships, sexually transmitted infections (STIs) and how to avoid them, and birth control methods.
Data collection	Data collection is a term used to describe a process of preparing and collecting data - for example as part of a process improvement or similar project. The purpose of Data collection is to obtain information to keep on record, to make decisions about important issues, to pass information on to others. Primarily, data is collected to provide information regarding a specific topic.
	Data collection usually takes place early on in an improvement project, and is often formalised through a Data collection plan which often contains the following activity.
	· Pre collection activity - Agree goals, target data, definitions, methods· Collection - Data collection· Present Findings - usually involves some form of sorting analysis and/or presentation.
Risk factor	A Risk factor is a variable associated with an increased risk of disease or infection. Risk factors are correlational and not necessarily causal, because correlation does not imply causation.

Chapter 6. Health Promotion and the Individual,

Cardiovascular disease	Cardiovascular disease or Cardiovascular diseases refers to the class of diseases that involve the heart or blood vessels (arteries and veins). While the term technically refers to any disease that affects the cardiovascular system (as used in MeSH), it is usually used to refer to those related to atherosclerosis (arterial disease). These conditions have similar causes, mechanisms, and treatments.

CHAPTER QUIZ: KEY TERMS, PEOPLE, PLACES, CONCEPTS

1. _____ is a term used to describe a process of preparing and collecting data - for example as part of a process improvement or similar project. The purpose of _____ is to obtain information to keep on record, to make decisions about important issues, to pass information on to others. Primarily, data is collected to provide information regarding a specific topic.

   _____ usually takes place early on in an improvement project, and is often formalised through a _____ plan which often contains the following activity.

   · Pre collection activity - Agree goals, target data, definitions, methods· Collection - _____· Present Findings - usually involves some form of sorting analysis and/or presentation.

   a. Bacteriophage
   b. Bottletop
   c. The Education of Shelby Knox
   d. Data collection

2. _____ has been defined by the World Health Organization's 2005 Bangkok Charter for _____ in a Globalized World as 'the process of enabling people to increase control over their health and its determinants, and thereby improve their health'. The primary means of _____ occur through developing healthy public policy that addresses the prerequisities of health such as income, housing, food security, employment, and quality working conditions. There is a tendency among public health officials and governments -- and this is especially the case in liberal nations such as Canada and the USA -- to reduce _____ to health education and social marketing focused on changing behavioral risk factors.

   a. Bacteriophage
   b. Baroreflex
   c. Benign prostatic hyperplasia
   d. Health promotion

3. . A _____ is a standardized statement about the health of a client (who can be an individual, a family, or a community) for the purpose of providing nursing care. Nursing diagnoses are developed based on data obtained during the nursing assessment.

The main organization for defining standard diagnoses in North America is the North American _____ Association, now known as NANDA-International.

a. abdominal exam
b. Nursing diagnosis
c. Acute HIV infection
d. Adenoviridae

4. _____ , refers to the treatment and management of illness, and the preservation of health through services offered by the medical, dental, complementary and alternative medicine, pharmaceutical, clinical laboratory sciences , nursing, and allied health professions. _____ embraces all the goods and services designed to promote health, including 'preventive, curative and palliative interventions, whether directed to individuals or to populations'.

Before the term _____ became popular, English-speakers referred to medicine or to the health sector and spoke of the treatment and prevention of illness and disease.

a. Bacteriophage
b. Health care
c. Benign prostatic hyperplasia
d. Benzathine benzylpenicillin

5. A _____ is a system to assess the severity of coma. There are several such systems:

The Glasgow _____ is neurological scale which aims to give a reliable, objective way of recording the conscious state of a person, for initial as well as continuing assessment. A patient is assessed against the criteria of the scale, and the resulting points give a patient score between 3 (indicating deep unconsciousness) and either 14 (original scale) or 15 (the more widely used modified or revised scale).

a. Bacteriophage
b. Baroreflex
c. Benign prostatic hyperplasia
d. Coma scale

1. d
2. d
3. b
4. b
5. d

You can take the complete Chapter Practice Test

for Chapter 6. Health Promotion and the Individual,
on all key terms, persons, places, and concepts.

Online 99 Cents

http://www.epub1625.32.20273.6.cram101.com/

Use www.Cram101.com for all your study needs

including Cram101's online interactive problem solving labs in

chemistry, statistics, mathematics, and more.

Chapter 7. Health Promotion and the Family,

_____ | Health promotion

_____ | Risk factor

_____ | Nuclear family

_____ | Child abuse

_____ | Elder abuse

_____ | Substance abuse

_____ | Nursing diagnosis

_____ | Genital wart

_____ | Community health

_____ | Health effect

_____ | Data collection

_____ | Genital herpes

_____ | Herpes simplex

_____ | Sexually transmitted disease

_____ | Case study

_____ | Health care

_____ | Lead poisoning

_____ | Health education

_____ | Alcohol abuse

CHAPTER OUTLINE: KEY TERMS, PEOPLE, PLACES, CONCEPTS

Communication

Adrenocorticotropic hormone

Family planning

CHAPTER HIGHLIGHTS & NOTES: KEY TERMS, PEOPLE, PLACES, CONCEPTS

Health promotion	Health promotion has been defined by the World Health Organization's 2005 Bangkok Charter for Health promotion in a Globalized World as 'the process of enabling people to increase control over their health and its determinants, and thereby improve their health'. The primary means of Health promotion occur through developing healthy public policy that addresses the prerequisities of health such as income, housing, food security, employment, and quality working conditions. There is a tendency among public health officials and governments -- and this is especially the case in liberal nations such as Canada and the USA -- to reduce Health promotion to health education and social marketing focused on changing behavioral risk factors.
Risk factor	A Risk factor is a variable associated with an increased risk of disease or infection. Risk factors are correlational and not necessarily causal, because correlation does not imply causation. For example, being young cannot be said to cause measles, but young people are more at risk as they are less likely to have developed immunity during a previous epidemic.
Nuclear family	A Nuclear family is a family group consisting of only a father and mother and their children, who share living quarters. This can be contrasted with an extended family. Nuclear families can be of any size, as long as there are only children and two parents.
Child abuse	Child abuse is the physical or psychological/emotional mistreatment of children. In the United States, the Centers for Disease Control and Prevention (CDC) define child maltreatment as any act or series of acts of commission or omission by a parent or other caregiver that results in harm, potential for harm, or threat of harm to a child. Most Child abuse occurs in a child's home, with a smaller amount occurring in the organizations, schools or communities the child interacts with.
Elder abuse	Elder abuse is a general term used to describe certain types of harm to older adults.

Chapter 7. Health Promotion and the Family,

Other terms commonly used include: 'elder mistreatment', 'senior abuse', 'abuse in later life', 'abuse of older adults', 'abuse of older women', and 'abuse of older men'.

One of the more commonly accepted definitions of Elder abuse is 'a single, or repeated act, or lack of appropriate action, occurring within any relationship where there is an expectation of trust which causes harm or distress to an older person.' This definition has been adopted by the World Health Organisation from a definition put forward by Action on Elder abuse in the UK.

The core feature of this definition is that it focuses on harms where there is 'expectation of trust' of the older person toward their abuser.

Substance abuse	Substance abuse also known as drug abuse, refers to a maladaptive pattern of use of a substance that is not considered dependent. The term 'drug abuse' does not exclude dependency, but is otherwise used in a similar manner in nonmedical contexts. The terms have a huge range of definitions related to taking a psychoactive drug or performance enhancing drug for a non-therapeutic or non-medical effect.
Nursing diagnosis	A Nursing diagnosis is a standardized statement about the health of a client (who can be an individual, a family, or a community) for the purpose of providing nursing care. Nursing diagnoses are developed based on data obtained during the nursing assessment. The main organization for defining standard diagnoses in North America is the North American Nursing diagnosis Association, now known as NANDA-International.
Genital wart	Genital warts (or Condylomata acuminata, venereal warts, anal warts and anogenital warts) is a highly contagious sexually transmitted disease caused by some sub-types of human papillomavirus (HPV). It is spread through direct skin-to-skin contact during oral, genital, or anal sex with an infected partner. Warts are the most easily recognized symptom of genital HPV infection, where types 6 and 11 are responsible for 90% of genital warts cases.
Community health	Community health, a field within public health, is a discipline that concerns itself with the study and betterment of the health characteristics of biological communities. While the term community can be broadly defined, Community health tends to focus on geographic areas rather than people with shared characteristics. The health characteristics of a community are often examined using geographic information system (GIS) software and public health datasets.
Health effect	Health effects are changes in health resulting from exposure to a source. Health effects are an important consideration in many areas, such as hygiene, pollution studies, workplace safety, nutrition and health sciences in general. Some of the major environmental sources of Health effects are air pollution, water pollution, soil contamination, noise pollution and over-illumination.

Data collection	Data collection is a term used to describe a process of preparing and collecting data - for example as part of a process improvement or similar project. The purpose of Data collection is to obtain information to keep on record, to make decisions about important issues, to pass information on to others. Primarily, data is collected to provide information regarding a specific topic.
	Data collection usually takes place early on in an improvement project, and is often formalised through a Data collection plan which often contains the following activity.
	· Pre collection activity - Agree goals, target data, definitions, methods· Collection - Data collection· Present Findings - usually involves some form of sorting analysis and/or presentation.
Genital herpes	Genital herpes refers to a genital infection by herpes simplex virus.
	Following the classification HSV into two distinct categories of HSV-1 and HSV-2 in the 1960s, it was established that 'HSV-2 was below the waist, HSV-1 was above the waist'. Although Genital herpes is largely believed to be caused by HSV-2, genital HSV-1 infections are increasing and now exceed 50% in certain populations, and that rule of thumb no longer applies.
Herpes simplex	Herpes simplex is a viral disease caused by both herpes simplex virus type 1 (HSV-1) and type 2 (HSV-2). Infection with the herpes virus is categorized into one of several distinct disorders based on the site of infection. Oral herpes, the visible symptoms of which are colloquially called cold sores or fever blisters, infects the face and mouth.
Sexually transmitted disease	A sexually transmitted disease also known as a sexually transmitted infection (STI), or venereal disease (VD), is an illness that has a significant probability of transmission between humans by means of human sexual behavior, including vaginal intercourse, oral sex, and anal sex. While in the past, these illnesses have mostly been referred to as Sexually transmitted diseases or VDs, in recent years the term sexually transmitted infections (STIs) has been preferred, as it has a broader range of meaning; a person may be infected, and may potentially infect others, without showing signs of disease. Some STIs can also be transmitted via the use of IV drug needles after its use by an infected person, as well as through childbirth or breastfeeding.
Case study	A Case study is a research methodology common in social science. It is based on an in-depth investigation of a single individual, group, or event to explore causation in order to find underlying principles.
Health care	Health care , refers to the treatment and management of illness, and the preservation of health through services offered by the medical, dental, complementary and alternative medicine, pharmaceutical, clinical laboratory sciences , nursing, and allied health professions.

Chapter 7. Health Promotion and the Family,

Health care embraces all the goods and services designed to promote health, including 'preventive, curative and palliative interventions, whether directed to individuals or to populations'.

Before the term Health care became popular, English-speakers referred to medicine or to the health sector and spoke of the treatment and prevention of illness and disease.

Lead poisoning	Lead poisoning is a medical condition caused by increased levels of the heavy metal lead in the body. Lead interferes with a variety of body processes and is toxic to many organs and tissues including the heart, bones, intestines, kidneys, and reproductive and nervous systems. It interferes with the development of the nervous system and is therefore particularly toxic to children, causing potentially permanent learning and behavior disorders.
Health education	Health education is the profession of educating people about health. Areas within this profession encompass environmental health, physical health, social health, emotional health, intellectual health, and spiritual health. It can be defined as the principle by which individuals and groups of people learn to behave in a manner conducive to the promotion, maintenance, or restoration of health.
Alcohol abuse	Alcohol abuse, as described in the DSM-IV, is a psychiatric diagnosis describing the recurring use of alcoholic beverages despite negative consequences. It is differentiated from alcohol dependence by the lack of symptoms such as tolerance and withdrawal. Alcohol abuse is sometimes referred to by the less specific term alcoholism.
Communication	Communication is a process of transferring information from one entity to another. Communication processes are sign-mediated interactions between at least two agents which share a repertoire of signs and semiotic rules. Communication is commonly defined as 'the imparting or interchange of thoughts, opinions, or information by speech, writing, or signs'.
Adrenocorticotropic hormone	Adrenocorticotropic hormone is a polypeptide tropic hormone produced and secreted by the anterior pituitary gland. It is an important component of the hypothalamic-pituitary-adrenal axis and is often produced in response to biological stress . Its principal effects are increased production of corticosteroids and, as its name suggests, cortisol from the adrenal cortex.
Family planning	Family planning is the planning of when to have children, and the use of birth control and other techniques to implement such plans. Other techniques commonly used include sexuality education, prevention and management of sexually transmitted infections, pre-conception counseling and management, and infertility management.

Chapter 7. Health Promotion and the Family,

1. _____s are changes in health resulting from exposure to a source. _____s are an important consideration in many areas, such as hygiene, pollution studies, workplace safety, nutrition and health sciences in general. Some of the major environmental sources of _____s are air pollution, water pollution, soil contamination, noise pollution and over-illumination.

   a. Health effector
   b. Blue Zone
   c. Health effect
   d. Deconditioning

2. _____ has been defined by the World Health Organization's 2005 Bangkok Charter for _____ in a Globalized World as 'the process of enabling people to increase control over their health and its determinants, and thereby improve their health'. The primary means of _____ occur through developing healthy public policy that addresses the prerequisites of health such as income, housing, food security, employment, and quality working conditions. There is a tendency among public health officials and governments -- and this is especially the case in liberal nations such as Canada and the USA -- to reduce _____ to health education and social marketing focused on changing behavioral risk factors.

   a. Bacteriophage
   b. Baroreflex
   c. Benign prostatic hyperplasia
   d. Health promotion

3. _____ is the planning of when to have children, and the use of birth control and other techniques to implement such plans. Other techniques commonly used include sexuality education, prevention and management of sexually transmitted infections, pre-conception counseling and management, and infertility management.

   _____ is sometimes used as a synonym for the use of birth control, though it often includes more.

   a. Family planning in India
   b. Guttmacher Institute
   c. Long-acting reversible contraceptive
   d. Family planning

4. _____ is a medical condition caused by increased levels of the heavy metal lead in the body. Lead interferes with a variety of body processes and is toxic to many organs and tissues including the heart, bones, intestines, kidneys, and reproductive and nervous systems. It interferes with the development of the nervous system and is therefore particularly toxic to children, causing potentially permanent learning and behavior disorders.

   a. Bacteriophage
   b. Lymphogranuloma venereum
   c. Lead poisoning
   d. Crede procedure

Chapter 7. Health Promotion and the Family,

5. _____, as described in the DSM-IV, is a psychiatric diagnosis describing the recurring use of alcoholic beverages despite negative consequences. It is differentiated from alcohol dependence by the lack of symptoms such as tolerance and withdrawal. _____ is sometimes referred to by the less specific term alcoholism.

    a. Alcohol withdrawal syndrome
    b. Alcohol dependence
    c. Alcohol abuse
    d. Alcoholic liver disease

ANSWER KEY
Chapter 7. Health Promotion and the Family,

1. c
2. d
3. d
4. c
5. c

You can take the complete Chapter Practice Test

for Chapter 7. Health Promotion and the Family,
on all key terms, persons, places, and concepts.

Online 99 Cents

http://www.epub1625.32.20273.7.cram101.com/

Use www.Cram101.com for all your study needs

including Cram101's online interactive problem solving labs in

chemistry, statistics, mathematics, and more.

CHAPTER OUTLINE: KEY TERMS, PEOPLE, PLACES, CONCEPTS

Health promotion

Community

Community health

Data collection

Risk factor

Interaction

Breast cancer

Case study

Guideline

Health care

Chapter 8. Health Promotion and the Community,

Health promotion	Health promotion has been defined by the World Health Organization's 2005 Bangkok Charter for Health promotion in a Globalized World as 'the process of enabling people to increase control over their health and its determinants, and thereby improve their health'. The primary means of Health promotion occur through developing healthy public policy that addresses the prerequisities of health such as income, housing, food security, employment, and quality working conditions. There is a tendency among public health officials and governments -- and this is especially the case in liberal nations such as Canada and the USA -- to reduce Health promotion to health education and social marketing focused on changing behavioral risk factors.
Community	In biological terms, a Community is a group of interacting organisms (or different species) sharing an environment. In human communities, intent, belief, resources, preferences, needs, risks, and a number of other conditions may be present and common, affecting the identity of the participants and their degree of cohesiveness. In sociology, the concept of Community has led to significant debate, and sociologists are yet to reach agreement on a definition of the term.
Community health	Community health, a field within public health, is a discipline that concerns itself with the study and betterment of the health characteristics of biological communities. While the term community can be broadly defined, Community health tends to focus on geographic areas rather than people with shared characteristics. The health characteristics of a community are often examined using geographic information system (GIS) software and public health datasets.
Data collection	Data collection is a term used to describe a process of preparing and collecting data - for example as part of a process improvement or similar project. The purpose of Data collection is to obtain information to keep on record, to make decisions about important issues, to pass information on to others. Primarily, data is collected to provide information regarding a specific topic. Data collection usually takes place early on in an improvement project, and is often formalised through a Data collection plan which often contains the following activity. · Pre collection activity - Agree goals, target data, definitions, methods· Collection - Data collection· Present Findings - usually involves some form of sorting analysis and/or presentation.
Risk factor	A Risk factor is a variable associated with an increased risk of disease or infection. Risk factors are correlational and not necessarily causal, because correlation does not imply causation. For example, being young cannot be said to cause measles, but young people are more at risk as they are less likely to have developed immunity during a previous epidemic.

Interaction	Interaction is a kind of action that occurs as two or more objects have an effect upon one another. The idea of a two-way effect is essential in the concept of Interaction, as opposed to a one-way causal effect. A closely related term is interconnectivity, which deals with the Interactions of Interactions within systems: combinations of many simple Interactions can lead to surprising emergent phenomena.
Breast cancer	Breast cancer is cancer originating from breast tissue, most commonly from the inner lining of milk ducts or the lobules that supply the ducts with milk. Cancers originating from ducts are known as ductal carcinomas; those originating from lobules are known as lobular carcinomas. The size, stage, rate of growth, and other characteristics of the tumor determine the kinds of treatment.
Case study	A Case study is a research methodology common in social science. It is based on an in-depth investigation of a single individual, group, or event to explore causation in order to find underlying principles.
Guideline	'Guideline' is the NATO reporting name for the Soviet SA-2 surface-to-air missile. A Guideline is any document that aims to streamline particular processes according to a set routine. By definition, following a Guideline is never mandatory (protocol would be a better term for a mandatory procedure).
Health care	Health care , refers to the treatment and management of illness, and the preservation of health through services offered by the medical, dental, complementary and alternative medicine, pharmaceutical, clinical laboratory sciences , nursing, and allied health professions. Health care embraces all the goods and services designed to promote health, including 'preventive, curative and palliative interventions, whether directed to individuals or to populations'. Before the term Health care became popular, English-speakers referred to medicine or to the health sector and spoke of the treatment and prevention of illness and disease.

Chapter 8. Health Promotion and the Community,

1. _____ is cancer originating from breast tissue, most commonly from the inner lining of milk ducts or the lobules that supply the ducts with milk. Cancers originating from ducts are known as ductal carcinomas; those originating from lobules are known as lobular carcinomas.

   The size, stage, rate of growth, and other characteristics of the tumor determine the kinds of treatment.

   a. Breast Cancer Action
   b. Breast cancer
   c. Breast Cancer Care
   d. Breast Cancer Research and Treatment

2. _____ has been defined by the World Health Organization's 2005 Bangkok Charter for _____ in a Globalized World as 'the process of enabling people to increase control over their health and its determinants, and thereby improve their health'. The primary means of _____ occur through developing healthy public policy that addresses the prerequisities of health such as income, housing, food security, employment, and quality working conditions. There is a tendency among public health officials and governments -- and this is especially the case in liberal nations such as Canada and the USA -- to reduce _____ to health education and social marketing focused on changing behavioral risk factors.

   a. Health promotion
   b. Baroreflex
   c. Benign prostatic hyperplasia
   d. Benzathine benzylpenicillin

3. A _____ is a variable associated with an increased risk of disease or infection. _____s are correlational and not necessarily causal, because correlation does not imply causation. For example, being young cannot be said to cause measles, but young people are more at risk as they are less likely to have developed immunity during a previous epidemic.

   a. Years of potential life lost
   b. Risk factor
   c. Late effect
   d. Bacteriophage

4. _____, a field within public health, is a discipline that concerns itself with the study and betterment of the health characteristics of biological communities. While the term community can be broadly defined, _____ tends to focus on geographic areas rather than people with shared characteristics. The health characteristics of a community are often examined using geographic information system (GIS) software and public health datasets.

   a. Bacteriophage
   b. Baroreflex
   c. Community health
   d. Benzathine benzylpenicillin

5. . In biological terms, a _____ is a group of interacting organisms (or different species) sharing an environment.

In human communities, intent, belief, resources, preferences, needs, risks, and a number of other conditions may be present and common, affecting the identity of the participants and their degree of cohesiveness.

In sociology, the concept of _____ has led to significant debate, and sociologists are yet to reach agreement on a definition of the term.

a. Bacteriophage
b. Community
c. Benign prostatic hyperplasia
d. Benzathine benzylpenicillin

1. b
2. a
3. b
4. c
5. b

You can take the complete Chapter Practice Test

for Chapter 8. Health Promotion and the Community,
on all key terms, persons, places, and concepts.

Online 99 Cents

http://www.epub1625.32.20273.8.cram101.com/

Use www.Cram101.com for all your study needs

including Cram101's online interactive problem solving labs in

chemistry, statistics, mathematics, and more.

CHAPTER OUTLINE: KEY TERMS, PEOPLE, PLACES, CONCEPTS

| | Case study |

| | Screening |

| | Health care |

| | Prevalence |

| | Data collection |

| | Health education |

| | Environmental health |

| | Risk factor |

| | Breast cancer |

| | Breast cancer screening |

| | Cancer screening |

| | Cervical |

| | Cervical cancer |

| | Colonoscopy |

| | Digestion |

| | Prostate cancer |

| | Cholesterol |

| | Colorectal cancer |

| | Prostate |

	Rectal examination

	Blood pressure

	Heart failure

	Hypertension

	Diabetes mellitus

	Diabetes

	Phenylketonuria

CHAPTER HIGHLIGHTS & NOTES: KEY TERMS, PEOPLE, PLACES, CONCEPTS

Case study

A Case study is a research methodology common in social science. It is based on an in-depth investigation of a single individual, group, or event to explore causation in order to find underlying principles.

Screening

One meaning of Screening is the investigation of a great number of something (for instance, people) looking for those with a particular problem or feature. For example at an airport many bags are screened by x-ray to try to detect any which may contain weapons or explosives, and people are screened by passing through a metal detector. If only part of a population is screened, Screening is equivalent to sampling in statistics.

Important cases of Screening include:

· Screening · Screening

Screening can also mean preventing access of something by some sort of barrier. Particular cases:

· Electromagnetic shielding in physics, the exclusion of electric, magnetic, or electromagnetic fields by a metallic screen or shield · In atomic physics and chemistry, the Screening effect or atomic shielding is the reduction of effective nuclear charge by intervening electron shells · Screening a process that represents lighter shades as tiny dots, rather than solid areas, of ink by passing ink through a perforated screen · The investigation of a large population is related; the members of a population are filtered by a metaphorical, rather than physical, screen · Screening is a process stage when cleaning paper pulp

Other uses:

· Film Screening, showing a film by projection onto a screen

Health care	Health care , refers to the treatment and management of illness, and the preservation of health through services offered by the medical, dental, complementary and alternative medicine, pharmaceutical, clinical laboratory sciences , nursing, and allied health professions. Health care embraces all the goods and services designed to promote health, including 'preventive, curative and palliative interventions, whether directed to individuals or to populations'. Before the term Health care became popular, English-speakers referred to medicine or to the health sector and spoke of the treatment and prevention of illness and disease.
Prevalence	In epidemiology, the Prevalence of a disease in a statistical population is defined as the total number of cases of the disease in the population at a given time divided by the number of individuals in the population. It is used as an estimate of how common a condition is within a population over a certain period of time. It helps physicians or other health professionals understand the probability of certain diagnoses and is routinely used by epidemiologists, health care providers, government agencies, and insurance companies.
Data collection	Data collection is a term used to describe a process of preparing and collecting data - for example as part of a process improvement or similar project. The purpose of Data collection is to obtain information to keep on record, to make decisions about important issues, to pass information on to others. Primarily, data is collected to provide information regarding a specific topic. Data collection usually takes place early on in an improvement project, and is often formalised through a Data collection plan which often contains the following activity. · Pre collection activity - Agree goals, target data, definitions, methods· Collection - Data collection· Present Findings - usually involves some form of sorting analysis and/or presentation.

Chapter 9. Screening,

Health education	Health education is the profession of educating people about health. Areas within this profession encompass environmental health, physical health, social health, emotional health, intellectual health, and spiritual health. It can be defined as the principle by which individuals and groups of people learn to behave in a manner conducive to the promotion, maintenance, or restoration of health.
Environmental health	Environmental health is the branch of public health that is concerned with all aspects of the natural and built environment that may affect human health. Other terms that refer to the discipline of Environmental health include environmental public health and Environmental health and protection. Environmental health is defined by the World Health Organization as:' Those aspects of human health and disease that are determined by factors in the environment.
Risk factor	A Risk factor is a variable associated with an increased risk of disease or infection. Risk factors are correlational and not necessarily causal, because correlation does not imply causation. For example, being young cannot be said to cause measles, but young people are more at risk as they are less likely to have developed immunity during a previous epidemic.
Breast cancer	Breast cancer is cancer originating from breast tissue, most commonly from the inner lining of milk ducts or the lobules that supply the ducts with milk. Cancers originating from ducts are known as ductal carcinomas; those originating from lobules are known as lobular carcinomas. The size, stage, rate of growth, and other characteristics of the tumor determine the kinds of treatment.
Breast cancer screening	Breast cancer screening refers to testing otherwise-healthy women for breast cancer in an attempt to achieve an earlier diagnosis. The assumption is that early detection will improve outcomes. A number of screening test have been employed including: clinical and self breast exams, mammography, genetic screening, ultrasound, and magnetic resonance imaging.
Cancer screening	Cancer screening occurs for many type of cancer including breast, prostate, lung, and colorectal cancer. Cancer screening is an attempt to detect unsuspected cancers in an asymptomatic population. Screening tests suitable for large numbers of healthy people must be relatively affordable, safe, noninvasive procedures with acceptably low rates of false positive results.If signs of cancer are detected, more definitive and invasive follow up tests are performed to confirm the diagnosis.
Cervical	In anatomy, 'Cervical' is an adjective that has two meanings:

· of or pertaining to any neck. · of or pertaining to the female cervix: i.e., the neck of the uterus.

· Commonly used medical phrases involving the neck are

· Cervical collar · Cervical disc (intervertebral disc) · Cervical lymph nodes · Cervical nerves · Cervical vertebrae · Cervical rib

· Phrases that involve the cervix include

· Cervical cancer · Cervical smear or Pap smear

Cervical cancer	Cervical cancer is malignant neoplasm of the cervix uteri or cervical area. It may present with vaginal bleeding, but symptoms may be absent until the cancer is in its advanced stages. Treatment consists of surgery (including local excision) in early stages and chemotherapy and radiotherapy in advanced stages of the disease.
Colonoscopy	Colonoscopy is the endoscopic examination of the colon and the distal part of the small bowel with a CCD camera or a fiber optic camera on a flexible tube passed through the anus. It may provide a visual diagnosis and grants the opportunity for biopsy or removal of suspected lesions. Virtual Colonoscopy, which uses 2D and 3D imagery reconstructed from computed tomography (CT) scans or from nuclear magnetic resonance (MR) scans, is also possible, as a totally non-invasive medical test, although it is not standard and still under investigation regarding its diagnostic abilities.
Digestion	Digestion is the mechanical and chemical breaking down of food into smaller components, to a form that can be absorbed, for instance, into a blood stream. Digestion is a form of catabolism; a break-down of macro food molecules to smaller ones. In mammals, food enters the mouth, being chewed by teeth, with chemical processing beginning with chemicals in the saliva from the salivary glands.
Prostate cancer	Prostate cancer is a form of cancer that develops in the prostate, a gland in the male reproductive system. The cancer cells may metastasize (spread) from the prostate to other parts of the body, particularly the bones and lymph nodes. Prostate cancer may cause pain, difficulty in urinating, problems during sexual intercourse, or erectile dysfunction.
Cholesterol	Cholesterol is a waxy steroid metabolite found in the cell membranes and transported in the blood plasma of all animals. It is an essential structural component of mammalian cell membranes, where it is required to establish proper membrane permeability and fluidity.

Chapter 9. Screening,

Colorectal cancer	Colorectal cancer, includes cancerous growths in the colon, rectum and appendix. With 655,000 deaths worldwide per year, it is the fourth most common form of cancer in the United States and the third leading cause of cancer-related death in the Western world. Colorectal cancers arise from adenomatous polyps in the colon.
Prostate	The Prostate is a compound tubuloalveolar exocrine gland of the male reproductive system in most mammals.
	In 2002, female paraurethral glands, or Skene's glands, were officially renamed the female Prostate by the Federative International Committee on Anatomical Terminology.
	The Prostate differs considerably among species anatomically, chemically, and physiologically.
Rectal examination	A Rectal examination or rectal exam is an internal examination of the rectum such as by a physician or other healthcare professional. Digital rectal exam: side view of the male reproductive and urinary anatomy, including the prostate, rectum, and bladder.
	The digital Rectal examination is a relatively simple procedure. The patient undresses, then is placed in a position where the anus is accessible .
Blood pressure	Blood pressure is the pressure (force per unit area) exerted by circulating blood on the walls of blood vessels, and constitutes one of the principal vital signs. The pressure of the circulating blood decreases as it moves away from the heart through arteries and capillaries, and toward the heart through veins. When unqualified, the term Blood pressure usually refers to brachial arterial pressure: that is, in the major blood vessel of the upper left or right arm that takes blood away from the heart.
Heart failure	Heart failure is generally defined as inability of the heart to supply sufficient blood flow to meet the body's needs. It has various diagnostic criteria, and the term heart failure is often incorrectly used to describe other cardiac-related illnesses, such as myocardial infarction (heart attack) or cardiac arrest.
	Common causes of heart failure include myocardial infarction (heart attacks) and other forms of ischemic heart disease, hypertension, valvular heart disease, and cardiomyopathy.
Hypertension	Hypertension or high blood pressure is a cardiac chronic medical condition in which the systemic arterial blood pressure is elevated. It is the opposite of hypotension. Hypertension is classified as either primary (essential) or secondary.
Diabetes mellitus	Diabetes mellitus strikes 1 in 400 cats and a similar number of dogs, though recent veterinary studies note that it is becoming more common lately in cats.

Symptoms in dogs and cats are similar to those in humans. Generally, most dogs and about 5-20% of cats experience type-1 (insulin-dependent) diabetes, rather than the type-2 that's now becoming common in obese humans.

Diabetes	diabetes mellitus --often referred to as diabetes--is a condition in which the body either does not produce enough, or does not properly respond to, insulin, a hormone produced in the pancreas. Insulin enables cells to absorb glucose in order to turn it into energy. This causes glucose to accumulate in the blood , leading to various potential complications. Many types of diabetes are recognized: The principal three are: · Type 1: Results from the body's failure to produce insulin.
Phenylketonuria	Phenylketonuria is an autosomal recessive metabolic genetic disorder characterized by a deficiency in the hepatic enzyme phenylalanine hydroxylase (PAH). This enzyme is necessary to metabolize the amino acid phenylalanine ('Phe') to the amino acid tyrosine. When PAH is deficient, phenylalanine accumulates and is converted into phenylpyruvate (also known as phenylketone), which is detected in the urine.

1. _____ is the profession of educating people about health. Areas within this profession encompass environmental health, physical health, social health, emotional health, intellectual health, and spiritual health. It can be defined as the principle by which individuals and groups of people learn to behave in a manner conducive to the promotion, maintenance, or restoration of health.

   a. Mahatma Gandhi Institute of Medical Sciences
   b. Health education
   c. Breastfeeding
   d. Mark Lester

2. A _____ is a research methodology common in social science. It is based on an in-depth investigation of a single individual, group, or event to explore causation in order to find underlying principles.

   a. Bacteriophage
   b. Baroreflex
   c. Benign prostatic hyperplasia
   d. Case study

Chapter 9. Screening,

3. _____ is cancer originating from breast tissue, most commonly from the inner lining of milk ducts or the lobules that supply the ducts with milk. Cancers originating from ducts are known as ductal carcinomas; those originating from lobules are known as lobular carcinomas.

   The size, stage, rate of growth, and other characteristics of the tumor determine the kinds of treatment.

   a. Breast Cancer Action
   b. Breast Cancer Campaign
   c. Breast Cancer Care
   d. Breast cancer

4. _____ strikes 1 in 400 cats and a similar number of dogs, though recent veterinary studies note that it is becoming more common lately in cats. Symptoms in dogs and cats are similar to those in humans. Generally, most dogs and about 5-20% of cats experience type-1 (insulin-dependent) diabetes, rather than the type-2 that's now becoming common in obese humans.

   a. abdominal exam
   b. Diabetes mellitus
   c. Myocardial infarction management
   d. NINCDS-ADRDA Alzheimer's Criteria

5. _____ is the branch of public health that is concerned with all aspects of the natural and built environment that may affect human health. Other terms that refer to the discipline of _____ include environmental public health and _____ and protection.

   _____ is defined by the World Health Organization as:'

   Those aspects of human health and disease that are determined by factors in the environment.

   a. Environmental health
   b. abdominal exam
   c. Achilles tendon
   d. Acute HIV infection

1. b
2. d
3. d
4. b
5. a

You can take the complete Chapter Practice Test

for Chapter 9. Screening,
on all key terms, persons, places, and concepts.

Online 99 Cents

http://www.epub1625.32.20273.9.cram101.com/

Use www.Cram101.com for all your study needs

including Cram101's online interactive problem solving labs in

chemistry, statistics, mathematics, and more.

	Health education
	Risk factor
	Nursing
	Health care
	Data collection
	Sex education
	Transtheoretical model
	Social marketing
	Cardiovascular disease
	Telenursing

Health education   Health education is the profession of educating people about health. Areas within this profession encompass environmental health, physical health, social health, emotional health, intellectual health, and spiritual health. It can be defined as the principle by which individuals and groups of people learn to behave in a manner conducive to the promotion, maintenance, or restoration of health.

Risk factor   A Risk factor is a variable associated with an increased risk of disease or infection. Risk factors are correlational and not necessarily causal, because correlation does not imply causation. For example, being young cannot be said to cause measles, but young people are more at risk as they are less likely to have developed immunity during a previous epidemic.

Chapter 10. Health Education,

Nursing	Nursing is a healthcare profession focused on the care of individuals, families, and communities so they may attain, maintain, or recover optimal health and quality of life from conception to death. Nurses work in a large variety of specialties where they work independently and as part of a team to assess, plan, implement and evaluate care. Nursing Science is a field of knowledge based on the contributions of nursing scientist through peer reviewed scholarly journals and evidenced-based practice.
Health care	Health care , refers to the treatment and management of illness, and the preservation of health through services offered by the medical, dental, complementary and alternative medicine, pharmaceutical, clinical laboratory sciences , nursing, and allied health professions. Health care embraces all the goods and services designed to promote health, including 'preventive, curative and palliative interventions, whether directed to individuals or to populations'. Before the term Health care became popular, English-speakers referred to medicine or to the health sector and spoke of the treatment and prevention of illness and disease.
Data collection	Data collection is a term used to describe a process of preparing and collecting data - for example as part of a process improvement or similar project. The purpose of Data collection is to obtain information to keep on record, to make decisions about important issues, to pass information on to others. Primarily, data is collected to provide information regarding a specific topic. Data collection usually takes place early on in an improvement project, and is often formalised through a Data collection plan which often contains the following activity. · Pre collection activity - Agree goals, target data, definitions, methods· Collection - Data collection· Present Findings - usually involves some form of sorting analysis and/or presentation.
Sex education	Sex education is a broad term used to describe education about human sexual anatomy, sexual reproduction, sexual intercourse, reproductive health, emotional relations, reproductive rights and responsibilities, abstinence, contraception, and other aspects of human sexual behavior. Common avenues for sex education are parents or caregivers, school programs, and public health campaigns. Overview

Chapter 10. Health Education,

Transtheoretical model	The Transtheoretical model in health psychology is intended to explain or predict a person's success or failure in achieving a proposed behavior change, such as developing different habits. It attempts to answer why the change 'stuck' or alternatively why the change was not made.
	The Transtheoretical model is also known by the acronym 'TTranstheoretical model' and by the term 'stages of change model'.
Social marketing	Social marketing is the systematic application of marketing, along with other concepts and techniques, to achieve specific behavioral goals for a social good. Social marketing can be applied to promote merit goods, or to make a society avoid demerit goods and thus to promote society's well being as a whole. For example, this may include asking people not to smoke in public areas, asking them to use seat belts, or prompting to make them follow speed limits.
Cardiovascular disease	Cardiovascular disease or Cardiovascular diseases refers to the class of diseases that involve the heart or blood vessels (arteries and veins). While the term technically refers to any disease that affects the cardiovascular system (as used in MeSH), it is usually used to refer to those related to atherosclerosis (arterial disease). These conditions have similar causes, mechanisms, and treatments.
Telenursing	Telenursing refers to the use of telecommunications and information technology for providing nursing services in health care whenever a large physical distance exists between patient and nurse, or between any number of nurses. As a field it is part of telehealth, and has many points of contacts with other medical and non-medical applications, such as telediagnosis, teleconsultation, telemonitoring, etc.
	Telenursing is achieving a large rate of growth in many countries, due to several factors: the preoccupation in driving down the costs of health care, an increase in the number of aging and chronically ill population, and the increase in coverage of health care to distant, rural, small or sparsely populated regions.

Chapter 10. Health Education,

1. _____ is a broad term used to describe education about human sexual anatomy, sexual reproduction, sexual intercourse, reproductive health, emotional relations, reproductive rights and responsibilities, abstinence, contraception, and other aspects of human sexual behavior. Common avenues for _____ are parents or caregivers, school programs, and public health campaigns.

   Overview

   _____ may also be described as 'sexuality education', which means that it encompasses education about all aspects of sexuality, including information about family planning, reproduction (fertilization, conception and development of the embryo and fetus, through to childbirth), plus information about all aspects of one's sexuality including: body image, sexual orientation, sexual pleasure, values, decision making, communication, dating, relationships, sexually transmitted infections (STIs) and how to avoid them, and birth control methods.

   a. Sex education
   b. Bottletop
   c. The Education of Shelby Knox
   d. Fistgate

2. _____ is a healthcare profession focused on the care of individuals, families, and communities so they may attain, maintain, or recover optimal health and quality of life from conception to death.

   Nurses work in a large variety of specialties where they work independently and as part of a team to assess, plan, implement and evaluate care. _____ Science is a field of knowledge based on the contributions of _____ scientist through peer reviewed scholarly journals and evidenced-based practice.

   a. Nutritionist
   b. Short-term exposure limit
   c. Nursing
   d. Baroreflex

3. A _____ is a variable associated with an increased risk of disease or infection. _____s are correlational and not necessarily causal, because correlation does not imply causation. For example, being young cannot be said to cause measles, but young people are more at risk as they are less likely to have developed immunity during a previous epidemic.

   a. Years of potential life lost
   b. Disease surveillance
   c. Late effect
   d. Risk factor

4. . _____ is a term used to describe a process of preparing and collecting data - for example as part of a process improvement or similar project. The purpose of _____ is to obtain information to keep on record, to make decisions about important issues, to pass information on to others. Primarily, data is collected to provide information regarding a specific topic.

_____ usually takes place early on in an improvement project, and is often formalised through a _____ plan which often contains the following activity.

· Pre collection activity - Agree goals, target data, definitions, methods· Collection - _____· Present Findings - usually involves some form of sorting analysis and/or presentation.

a. Bacteriophage
b. Data collection
c. Baroreflex
d. Benign prostatic hyperplasia

5. _____ or _____s refers to the class of diseases that involve the heart or blood vessels (arteries and veins). While the term technically refers to any disease that affects the cardiovascular system (as used in MeSH), it is usually used to refer to those related to atherosclerosis (arterial disease). These conditions have similar causes, mechanisms, and treatments.

a. Bacteriophage
b. Cardiovascular disease
c. The Education of Shelby Knox
d. Fistgate

1. a
2. c
3. d
4. b
5. b

You can take the complete Chapter Practice Test

for Chapter 10. Health Education,
on all key terms, persons, places, and concepts.

Online 99 Cents

http://www.epub1625.32.20273.10.cram101.com/

Use www.Cram101.com for all your study needs

including Cram101's online interactive problem solving labs in

chemistry, statistics, mathematics, and more.

Chapter 11. Nutrition Counseling for Health Promotion,

CHAPTER OUTLINE: KEY TERMS, PEOPLE, PLACES, CONCEPTS

Health promotion

Life expectancy

Childhood obesity

Blood pressure

Case study

Dietary Reference Intake

Toilet training

Fatty acid

Prescription drug

Food safety

Vitamin D

Vitamin E

Adverse effect

Nutrition

Toxicity

Bovine spongiform encephalopathy

Salmonellosis

Avian influenza

Cardiovascular disease

CHAPTER OUTLINE: KEY TERMS, PEOPLE, PLACES, CONCEPTS

	Malnutrition
	Screening
	Low-density lipoprotein
	National Cholesterol Education Program
	Risk factor
	Good cholesterol
	Metabolic syndrome
	Health education
	Epidemiology
	Hypertension
	American Cancer Society
	Sodium chloride
	Cancer
	Osteoporosis
	Pathophysiology
	Body mass index
	Weight loss
	Growth chart
	Prevalence

Chapter 11. Nutrition Counseling for Health Promotion,

CHAPTER OUTLINE: KEY TERMS, PEOPLE, PLACES. CONCEPTS

Diabetes

Breast self-examination

CHAPTER HIGHLIGHTS & NOTES: KEY TERMS, PEOPLE, PLACES, CONCEPTS

Health promotion	Health promotion has been defined by the World Health Organization's 2005 Bangkok Charter for Health promotion in a Globalized World as 'the process of enabling people to increase control over their health and its determinants, and thereby improve their health'. The primary means of Health promotion occur through developing healthy public policy that addresses the prerequisities of health such as income, housing, food security, employment, and quality working conditions. There is a tendency among public health officials and governments -- and this is especially the case in liberal nations such as Canada and the USA -- to reduce Health promotion to health education and social marketing focused on changing behavioral risk factors.
Life expectancy	Life expectancy is the average number of years of life remaining at a given age. The term is most often used in the human context, but used also in plant or animal ecology and the calculation is based on the analysis of life tables (also known as actuarial tables). The term may also be used in the context of manufactured objects although the related term shelf life is used for consumer products and the term mean time to breakdown (MTTB) is used in engineering literature.
Childhood obesity	Childhood obesity is a condition where excess body fat negatively affects a child's health or wellbeing. As methods to determine body fat directly are difficult, the diagnosis of obesity is often based on BMI. Due to the rising prevalence of obesity in children and its many adverse health effects it is being recognized as a serious public health concern. The term overweight rather than obese is often used in children as it is less stigmatizing.
Blood pressure	Blood pressure is the pressure (force per unit area) exerted by circulating blood on the walls of blood vessels, and constitutes one of the principal vital signs. The pressure of the circulating blood decreases as it moves away from the heart through arteries and capillaries, and toward the heart through veins. When unqualified, the term Blood pressure usually refers to brachial arterial pressure: that is, in the major blood vessel of the upper left or right arm that takes blood away from the heart.
Case study	A Case study is a research methodology common in social science.

Visit Cram101.com for full Practice Exams

Dietary Reference Intake	The Dietary Reference Intake is a system of nutrition recommendations from the Institute of Medicine (IOM) of the U.S. National Academy of Sciences. The Dietary Reference Intake system is used by both the United States and Canada and is intended for the general public and health professionals. Applications include: · Composition of diets for schools, prisons, hospitals or nursing homes · Industries developing new food stuffs · Healthcare policy makers and public health officials The Dietary Reference Intake was introduced in 1997 in order to broaden the existing guidelines known as Recommended Dietary Allowances (RDAs). The Dietary Reference Intake values are not currently used in nutrition labeling, where the older Reference Daily Intake are still used.
Toilet training	Toilet training, or potty training, is the process of training a young child to use the toilet for urination and defecation, though training may start with a smaller toilet bowl-shaped device (often known as a potty). In Western countries it is usually started and completed between the ages of 12 months and three years with boys typically being at the higher end of the age spectrum. Cultural factors play a large part in what age is deemed appropriate, with the age being generally later in America. Most advise that Toilet training is a mutual task, requiring cooperation, agreement and understanding between child and the caregiver, and the best potty training techniques emphasize consistency and positive reinforcement over punishment - making it fun for the child.
Fatty acid	In chemistry, especially biochemistry, a fatty acid is a carboxylic acid often with a long unbranched aliphatic tail (chain), which is either saturated or unsaturated. Carboxylic acids as short as butyric acid (4 carbon atoms) are considered to be fatty acids, whereas fatty acids derived from natural fats and oils may be assumed to have at least eight carbon atoms, caprylic acid (octanoic acid), for example. The most abundant natural fatty acids have an even number of carbon atoms because their biosynthesis involves acetyl-CoA, a coenzyme carrying a two-carbon-atom group .
Prescription drug	A Prescription drug is a licensed medicine that is regulated by legislation to require a prescription before it can be obtained. The term is used to distinguish it from over-the-counter drugs which can be obtained without a prescription. Different jurisdictions have different definitions of what constitutes a Prescription drug.
Food safety	Food safety is a scientific discipline describing handling, preparation, and storage of food in ways that prevent foodborne illness. This includes a number of routines that should be followed to avoid potentially severe health hazards.

Vitamin D	Vitamin D is a group of fat-soluble prohormones, the two major forms of which are Vitamin D_2 (or ergocalciferol) and Vitamin D_3 (or cholecalciferol). Vitamin D obtained from sun exposure, food, and supplements, is biologically inert and must undergo two hydroxylation reactions to be activated in the body. Calcitriol (1,25-Dihydroxycholecalciferol) is the active form of Vitamin D found in the body.
Vitamin E	Vitamin E is a generic term for tocopherols and tocotrienols. Vitamin E is a family of α-, β-, γ-, and δ-tocopherols and corresponding four tocotrienols. Vitamin E is a fat-soluble antioxidant that stops the production of reactive oxygen species formed when fat undergoes oxidation.
Adverse effect	In medicine, an Adverse effect is a harmful and undesired effect resulting from a medication or other intervention such as surgery. An Adverse effect may be termed a 'side effect', when judged to be secondary to a main or therapeutic effect, and may result from an unsuitable or incorrect dosage or procedure, which could be due to medical error. Adverse effects are sometimes referred to as 'iatrogenic' because they are generated by a physician/treatment.
Nutrition	Nutrition is the provision, to cells and organisms, of the materials necessary (in the form of food) to support life. Many common health problems can be prevented or alleviated with a healthy diet. The diet of an organism is what it eats, and is largely determined by the perceived palatability of foods.
Toxicity	Toxicity is the degree to which a substance is able to damage an exposed organism. Toxicity can refer to the effect on a whole organism, such as an animal, bacterium, or plant, as well as the effect on a substructure of the organism, such as a cell (cytoToxicity) or an organ (organoToxicity), such as the liver (hepatoToxicity). By extension, the word may be metaphorically used to describe toxic effects on larger and more complex groups, such as the family unit or society at large.
Bovine spongiform encephalopathy	Mad Cow redirects here. wikimedia.org/wikipedia/commons/thumb/9/95/Aphis.usda.gov_Bovine spongiform encephalopathy_3.jpg/250px-Aphis.usda.gov_Bovine spongiform encephalopathy_3.jpg' width='250' height='200' /> Bovine spongiform encephalopathy commonly known as mad-cow disease, is a fatal neurodegenerative disease in cattle that causes a spongy degeneration in the brain and spinal cord. Bovine spongiform encephalopathy has a long incubation period, about 30 months to 8 years, usually affecting adult cattle at a peak age onset of four to five years, all breeds being equally susceptible.
Salmonellosis	Salmonellosis is an infection with Salmonella bacteria. Most people infected with Salmonella develop diarrhea, fever, vomiting, and abdominal cramps 8 to 72 hours after infection.

Avian influenza	Avian influenza, and commonly bird flu, refers to 'influenza caused by viruses adapted to birds.' Of the greatest concern is highly pathogenic avian influenza.

'Bird flu' is a phrase similar to 'swine flu,' 'dog flu,' 'horse flu,' or 'human flu' in that it refers to an illness caused by any of many different strains of influenza viruses that have adapted to a specific host. All known viruses that cause influenza in birds belong to the species influenza A virus. |
| Cardiovascular disease | Cardiovascular disease or Cardiovascular diseases refers to the class of diseases that involve the heart or blood vessels (arteries and veins). While the term technically refers to any disease that affects the cardiovascular system (as used in MeSH), it is usually used to refer to those related to atherosclerosis (arterial disease). These conditions have similar causes, mechanisms, and treatments. |
| Malnutrition | Malnutrition is the insufficient, excessive or imbalanced consumption of nutrients. A number of different nutrition disorders may arise, depending on which nutrients are under or overabundant in the diet.

The World Health Organization cites Malnutrition as the gravest single threat to the world's public health. |
| Screening | One meaning of Screening is the investigation of a great number of something (for instance, people) looking for those with a particular problem or feature. For example at an airport many bags are screened by x-ray to try to detect any which may contain weapons or explosives, and people are screened by passing through a metal detector. If only part of a population is screened, Screening is equivalent to sampling in statistics.

Important cases of Screening include:

· Screening · Screening

Screening can also mean preventing access of something by some sort of barrier. Particular cases:

· Electromagnetic shielding in physics, the exclusion of electric, magnetic, or electromagnetic fields by a metallic screen or shield · In atomic physics and chemistry, the Screening effect or atomic shielding is the reduction of effective nuclear charge by intervening electron shells · Screening a process that represents lighter shades as tiny dots, rather than solid areas, of ink by passing ink through a perforated screen · The investigation of a large population is related; the members of a population are filtered by a metaphorical, rather than physical, screen · Screening is a process stage when cleaning paper pulp |

Chapter 11. Nutrition Counseling for Health Promotion,

Other uses:

· Film Screening, showing a film by projection onto a screen

Low-density lipoprotein	Low-density lipoprotein is a type of lipoprotein that transports cholesterol and triglycerides from the liver to peripheral tissues. LDL is one of the five major groups of lipoproteins; these groups include chylomicrons, very Low-density lipoprotein intermediate-density lipoprotein (IDL), Low-density lipoprotein, and high-density lipoprotein (HDL), although some alternative organizational schemes have been proposed. Like all lipoproteins, LDL enables fats and cholesterol to move within the water-based solution of the blood stream.
National Cholesterol Education Program	The National Cholesterol Education Program is a program managed by the National Heart, Lung and Blood Institute, a division of the National Institutes of Health. Its goal is to reduce increased cardiovascular disease rates due to hypercholesterolemia (elevated cholesterol levels) in the United States of America. The program has been running since 1985.

The assigned goal of the National Cholesterol Education Program committee is to meet on a recurring basis, review ongoing scientific research about atherosclerotic cardiovascular disease and make simplified, consensus, committee recommendations to be promoted by the NIH, the American Heart Association and other groups to both physicians and the public about how to reduce the incidence of disability and death resulting from atherosclerotic cardiovascular disease. |
| Risk factor | A Risk factor is a variable associated with an increased risk of disease or infection. Risk factors are correlational and not necessarily causal, because correlation does not imply causation. For example, being young cannot be said to cause measles, but young people are more at risk as they are less likely to have developed immunity during a previous epidemic. |
| Good cholesterol | High-density lipoprotein is one of the five major groups of lipoproteins (chylomicrons, VLDL, IDL, LDL, HDL) that enable lipids like cholesterol and triglycerides to be transported within the water-based bloodstream. In healthy individuals, about thirty percent of blood cholesterol is carried by HDL.

It is hypothesized that HDL can remove cholesterol from atheroma within arteries and transport it back to the liver for excretion or re-utilization, which is the main reason why HDL-bound cholesterol is sometimes called 'good cholesterol', or HDL-C. A high level of HDL-C seems to protect against cardiovascular diseases, and low HDL cholesterol levels (less than 40 mg/dL or about 1mmol/L) increase the risk for heart disease. Cholesterol contained in HDL particles is considered beneficial for the cardiovascular health, in contrast to 'bad' LDL cholesterol. |

Metabolic syndrome	Metabolic syndrome is a combination of medical disorders that, when occurring together, increase the risk of developing cardiovascular disease and diabetes. It affects one in five people in the United States and prevalence increases with age. Some studies have shown the prevalence in the USA to be an estimated 25% of the population.
Health education	Health education is the profession of educating people about health. Areas within this profession encompass environmental health, physical health, social health, emotional health, intellectual health, and spiritual health. It can be defined as the principle by which individuals and groups of people learn to behave in a manner conducive to the promotion, maintenance, or restoration of health.
Epidemiology	Epidemiology is the study of factors affecting the health and illness of populations, and serves as the foundation and logic of interventions made in the interest of public health and preventive medicine. It is considered a cornerstone methodology of public health research, and is highly regarded in evidence-based medicine for identifying risk factors for disease and determining optimal treatment approaches to clinical practice. In the study of communicable and non-communicable diseases, the work of epidemiologists ranges from outbreak investigation to study design, data collection and analysis including the development of statistical models to test hypotheses and the documentation of results for submission to peer-reviewed journals.
Hypertension	Hypertension or high blood pressure is a cardiac chronic medical condition in which the systemic arterial blood pressure is elevated. It is the opposite of hypotension. Hypertension is classified as either primary (essential) or secondary.
American Cancer Society	The American Cancer Society is the 'nationwide community-based voluntary health organization dedicated to eliminating cancer as a major health problem by preventing cancer, saving lives, and diminishing suffering from cancer, through research, education, advocacy and service.' The society is organized into thirteen geographical divisions of both medical and lay volunteers operating in more than 3,400 offices throughout the United States and Puerto Rico. Its home office is located in the American Cancer Society Center in Atlanta, Georgia. As its official journal the American Cancer Society publishes Cancer.
Sodium chloride	Sodium chloride, also known as common salt, table salt is an ionic compound with the formula NaCl. Sodium chloride is the salt most responsible for the salinity of the ocean and of the extracellular fluid of many multicellular organisms. As the major ingredient in edible salt, it is commonly used as a condiment and food preservative.
Cancer	Cancer (medical term: malignant neoplasm) is a class of diseases in which a group of cells display uncontrolled growth, invasion that intrudes upon and destroys adjacent tissues, and sometimes metastasis, or spreading to other locations in the body via lymph or blood.

	These three malignant properties of cancers differentiate them from benign tumors, which do not invade or metastasize.
	Researchers divide the causes of cancer into two groups: those with an environmental cause and those with a hereditary genetic cause.
Osteoporosis	Osteoporosis is a disease of bones that leads to an increased risk of fracture. In osteoporosis the bone mineral density (BMD) is reduced, bone microarchitecture deteriorates, and the amount and variety of proteins in bone is altered. Osteoporosis is defined by the World Health Organization (WHO) as a bone mineral density that is 2.5 standard deviations or more below the mean peak bone mass (average of young, healthy adults) as measured by DXA; the term 'established osteoporosis' includes the presence of a fragility fracture.
Pathophysiology	Pathophysiology is the study of the changes of normal mechanical, physical, and biochemical functions, either caused by a disease, or resulting from an abnormal syndrome. More formally, it is the branch of medicine which deals with any disturbances of body functions, caused by disease or prodromal symptoms.
	An alternate definition is 'the study of the biological and physical manifestations of disease as they correlate with the underlying abnormalities and physiological disturbances.'
	The study of pathology and the study of Pathophysiology often involves substantial overlap in diseases and processes, but pathology emphasizes direct observations, while Pathophysiology emphasizes quantifiable measurements.
Body mass index	The Body mass index is a controversial statistical measurement which compares a person's weight and height. Though it does not actually measure the percentage of body fat, it may be a useful tool to estimate a healthy body weight based on how tall a person is. Due to its ease of measurement and calculation, it is the most widely used diagnostic tool to identify weight problems within a population, usually whether individuals are underweight, overweight or obese.
Weight loss	Weight loss, in the context of medicine, health or physical fitness, is a reduction of the total body mass, due to a mean loss of fluid, body fat or adipose tissue and/or lean mass, namely bone mineral deposits, muscle, tendon and other connective tissue. It can occur unintentionally due to an underlying disease or can arise from a conscious effort to improve an actual or perceived overweight or obese state.
	Unintentional weight loss

Growth chart	A Growth chart is used by pediatricians and other health care providers to follow a child's growth over time. Growth charts have been constructed by observing the growth of large numbers of normal children over time. The height, weight, and head circumference of a child can be compared to the expected parameters of children of the same age and sex to determine whether the child is growing appropriately.
Prevalence	In epidemiology, the Prevalence of a disease in a statistical population is defined as the total number of cases of the disease in the population at a given time divided by the number of individuals in the population. It is used as an estimate of how common a condition is within a population over a certain period of time. It helps physicians or other health professionals understand the probability of certain diagnoses and is routinely used by epidemiologists, health care providers, government agencies, and insurance companies.
Diabetes	diabetes mellitus --often referred to as diabetes--is a condition in which the body either does not produce enough, or does not properly respond to, insulin, a hormone produced in the pancreas. Insulin enables cells to absorb glucose in order to turn it into energy. This causes glucose to accumulate in the blood , leading to various potential complications. Many types of diabetes are recognized: The principal three are: · Type 1: Results from the body's failure to produce insulin.
Breast self-examination	Breast self-examination (Breast self-examinationE) is a method of finding abnormalities of the breast, for early detection of breast cancer. The method involves the woman herself looking at and feeling each breast for possible lumps, distortions or swelling. Breast self-examinationE was once promoted heavily as a means of finding cancer at a more curable stage, but randomized controlled studies found that it was not effective in preventing death, and actually caused harm through needless biopsies and surgery.

Chapter 11. Nutrition Counseling for Health Promotion,

1. _____ is a combination of medical disorders that, when occurring together, increase the risk of developing cardiovascular disease and diabetes. It affects one in five people in the United States and prevalence increases with age. Some studies have shown the prevalence in the USA to be an estimated 25% of the population.

   a. MORM syndrome
   b. Coloboma of optic nerve
   c. Mungan Syndrome
   d. Metabolic syndrome

2. _____ is the pressure (force per unit area) exerted by circulating blood on the walls of blood vessels, and constitutes one of the principal vital signs. The pressure of the circulating blood decreases as it moves away from the heart through arteries and capillaries, and toward the heart through veins. When unqualified, the term _____ usually refers to brachial arterial pressure: that is, in the major blood vessel of the upper left or right arm that takes blood away from the heart.

   a. Korotkoff
   b. Blood pressure
   c. Bacteriophage
   d. Baroreflex

3. _____ is a condition where excess body fat negatively affects a child's health or wellbeing. As methods to determine body fat directly are difficult, the diagnosis of obesity is often based on BMI. Due to the rising prevalence of obesity in children and its many adverse health effects it is being recognized as a serious public health concern. The term overweight rather than obese is often used in children as it is less stigmatizing.

   a. Bacteriophage
   b. Childhood obesity
   c. Benign prostatic hyperplasia
   d. Benzathine benzylpenicillin

4. In epidemiology, the _____ of a disease in a statistical population is defined as the total number of cases of the disease in the population at a given time divided by the number of individuals in the population. It is used as an estimate of how common a condition is within a population over a certain period of time. It helps physicians or other health professionals understand the probability of certain diagnoses and is routinely used by epidemiologists, health care providers, government agencies, and insurance companies.

   a. Years of potential life lost
   b. Prevalence
   c. Late effect
   d. Bacteriophage

5. . In medicine, an _____ is a harmful and undesired effect resulting from a medication or other intervention such as surgery. An _____ may be termed a 'side effect', when judged to be secondary to a main or therapeutic effect, and may result from an unsuitable or incorrect dosage or procedure, which could be due to medical error. _____s are sometimes referred to as 'iatrogenic' because they are generated by a physician/treatment.

a. Elective surgery

b. Adverse effect

c. Extracorporeal

d. Agonist

1. d
2. b
3. b
4. b
5. b

You can take the complete Chapter Practice Test

for Chapter 11. Nutrition Counseling for Health Promotion,
on all key terms, persons, places, and concepts.

Online 99 Cents

http://www.epub1625.32.20273.11.cram101.com/

Use www.Cram101.com for all your study needs

including Cram101's online interactive problem solving labs in

chemistry, statistics, mathematics, and more.

CHAPTER OUTLINE: KEY TERMS, PEOPLE, PLACES, CONCEPTS

Cardiorespiratory fitness

Case study

Musculoskeletal system

Cardiovascular disease

Malnutrition

Good cholesterol

Hypertriglyceridemia

Lipid metabolism

Lipoprotein lipase

Risk factor

Resistance training

Hypertension

Prevalence

Osteoporosis

Prevention

Osteoarthritis

Rheumatoid arthritis

Arthritis

Back pain

Mental health

Respiratory tract

Breast cancer

Health economics

Prostate cancer

Cross-training

Heart rate

Exercise intensity

Water activity

Health care

Stretching

Diaphragmatic breathing

Diabetes mellitus

Rhythm

Data collection

Cardiorespiratory fitness	Cardiorespiratory fitness refers to the ability of the circulatory and respiratory systems to supply oxygen to skeletal muscles during sustained physical activity. Regular exercise makes these systems more efficient by enlarging the heart muscle, enabling more blood to be pumped with each stroke, and increasing the number of small arteries in trained skeletal muscles, which supply more blood to working muscles. Exercise improves the respiratory system by increasing the amount of oxygen that is inhaled and distributed to body tissues.
Case study	A Case study is a research methodology common in social science. It is based on an in-depth investigation of a single individual, group, or event to explore causation in order to find underlying principles.
Musculoskeletal system	A Musculoskeletal system is an organ system that gives animals (including humans) the ability to move using the muscular and skeletal systems. The Musculoskeletal system provides form, stability, and movement to the body. It is made up of the body's bones (the skeleton), muscles, cartilage, tendons, ligaments, joints, and other connective tissue (the tissue that supports and binds tissues and organs together).
Cardiovascular disease	Cardiovascular disease or Cardiovascular diseases refers to the class of diseases that involve the heart or blood vessels (arteries and veins). While the term technically refers to any disease that affects the cardiovascular system (as used in MeSH), it is usually used to refer to those related to atherosclerosis (arterial disease). These conditions have similar causes, mechanisms, and treatments.
Malnutrition	Malnutrition is the insufficient, excessive or imbalanced consumption of nutrients. A number of different nutrition disorders may arise, depending on which nutrients are under or overabundant in the diet. The World Health Organization cites Malnutrition as the gravest single threat to the world's public health.
Good cholesterol	High-density lipoprotein is one of the five major groups of lipoproteins (chylomicrons, VLDL, IDL, LDL, HDL) that enable lipids like cholesterol and triglycerides to be transported within the water-based bloodstream. In healthy individuals, about thirty percent of blood cholesterol is carried by HDL. It is hypothesized that HDL can remove cholesterol from atheroma within arteries and transport it back to the liver for excretion or re-utilization, which is the main reason why HDL-bound cholesterol is sometimes called 'good cholesterol', or HDL-C. A high level of HDL-C seems to protect against cardiovascular diseases, and low HDL cholesterol levels (less than 40 mg/dL or about 1mmol/L) increase the risk for heart disease.

Chapter 12. Exercise,

Hypertriglyceridemia	In medicine, Hypertriglyceridemia denotes high (hyper-) blood levels (-emia) of triglycerides, the most abundant fatty molecule in most organisms. It has been associated with atherosclerosis, even in the absence of hypercholesterolemia (high cholesterol levels). It can also lead to pancreatitis in excessive concentrations.
Lipid metabolism	Lipid metabolism refers to the processes that involve the creation and degradation of lipids.

The types of lipids involved include:

· bile salts · cholesterols · eicosanoids · glycolipids · ketone bodies · fatty acids · phospholipids · sphingolipids · steroid · triacylglycerols |
| Lipoprotein lipase | Lipoprotein lipase is an enzyme that hydrolyzes lipids in lipoproteins, such as those found in chylomicrons and very low-density lipoproteins (VLDL), into two free fatty acids and one monoacylglycerol molecule. It requires Apo-CII as a cofactor.

Lipoprotein lipase is specifically found in endothelial cells lining the capillaries. |
Risk factor	A Risk factor is a variable associated with an increased risk of disease or infection. Risk factors are correlational and not necessarily causal, because correlation does not imply causation. For example, being young cannot be said to cause measles, but young people are more at risk as they are less likely to have developed immunity during a previous epidemic.
Resistance training	Resistance training has two different meanings.
Hypertension	Hypertension or high blood pressure is a cardiac chronic medical condition in which the systemic arterial blood pressure is elevated. It is the opposite of hypotension. Hypertension is classified as either primary (essential) or secondary.
Prevalence	In epidemiology, the Prevalence of a disease in a statistical population is defined as the total number of cases of the disease in the population at a given time divided by the number of individuals in the population. It is used as an estimate of how common a condition is within a population over a certain period of time. It helps physicians or other health professionals understand the probability of certain diagnoses and is routinely used by epidemiologists, health care providers, government agencies, and insurance companies.
Osteoporosis	Osteoporosis is a disease of bones that leads to an increased risk of fracture. In osteoporosis the bone mineral density (BMD) is reduced, bone microarchitecture deteriorates, and the amount and variety of proteins in bone is altered.

Prevention	Prevention refers to: · Preventive medicine · Hazard Prevention, the process of risk study and elimination and mitigation in emergency management · Risk Prevention · Risk management · Preventive maintenance · Crime Prevention · Prevention, an album by Scottish band De Rosa · Prevention a magazine about health in the United States · Prevent (company), a textile company from Slovenia
Osteoarthritis	Osteoarthritis is a group of diseases and mechanical abnormalities involving degradation of joints, including articular cartilage and the subchondral bone next to it. Clinical manifestations of OA may include joint pain, tenderness, stiffness, creaking, locking of joints, and sometimes local inflammation. In OA, a variety of potential forces--hereditary, developmental, metabolic, and mechanical--may initiate processes leading to loss of cartilage -- a strong protein matrix that lubricates and cushions the joints.
Rheumatoid arthritis	Rheumatoid arthritis is a chronic, systemic inflammatory disorder that may affect many tissues and organs, but principally attacks the joints producing an inflammatory synovitis that often progresses to destruction of the articular cartilage and ankylosis of the joints. Rheumatoid arthritis can also produce diffuse inflammation in the lungs, pericardium, pleura, and sclera, and also nodular lesions, most common in subcutaneous tissue under the skin. Although the cause of Rheumatoid arthritis is unknown, autoimmunity plays a pivotal role in its chronicity and progression.
Arthritis	Arthritis is a group of conditions involving damage to the joints of the body. There are over 100 different forms of arthritis. The most common form, osteoarthritis is a result of trauma to the joint, infection of the joint, or age.
Back pain	Back pain (also known 'dorsalgia') is pain felt in the back that usually originates from the muscles, nerves, bones, joints or other structures in the spine. The pain can often be divided into neck pain, upper Back pain, lower Back pain or tailbone pain. It may have a sudden onset or can be a chronic pain; it can be constant or intermittent, stay in one place or radiate to other areas.
Mental health	Mental health is a term used to describe either a level of cognitive or emotional well-being or an absence of a mental disorder. From perspectives of the discipline of positive psychology or holism Mental health may include an individual's ability to enjoy life and procure a balance between life activities and efforts to achieve psychological resilience.

Chapter 12. Exercise,

Respiratory tract	In humans the Respiratory tract is the part of the anatomy that has to do with the process of respiration. The Respiratory tract is divided into 3 segments: · Upper Respiratory tract: nose and nasal passages, paranasal sinuses, and throat or pharynx · Respiratory airways: voice box or larynx, trachea, bronchi, and bronchioles · Lungs: respiratory bronchioles, alveolar ducts, alveolar sacs, and alveoli The Respiratory tract is a common site for infections. Upper Respiratory tract infections are probably the most common infections in the world. Most of the Respiratory tract exists merely as a piping system for air to travel in the lungs; alveoli are the only part of the lung that exchanges oxygen and carbon dioxide with the blood.
Breast cancer	Breast cancer is cancer originating from breast tissue, most commonly from the inner lining of milk ducts or the lobules that supply the ducts with milk. Cancers originating from ducts are known as ductal carcinomas; those originating from lobules are known as lobular carcinomas. The size, stage, rate of growth, and other characteristics of the tumor determine the kinds of treatment.
Health economics	Health economics is a branch of economics concerned with issues related to scarcity in the allocation of health and health care. For example, it is now clear that medical debt is the principle cause of bankruptcy in the United States. In broad terms, health economists study the functioning of the health care system and the private and social causes of health-affecting behaviors such as smoking.
Prostate cancer	Prostate cancer is a form of cancer that develops in the prostate, a gland in the male reproductive system. The cancer cells may metastasize (spread) from the prostate to other parts of the body, particularly the bones and lymph nodes. Prostate cancer may cause pain, difficulty in urinating, problems during sexual intercourse, or erectile dysfunction.
Cross-training	Cross-training refers to training in different ways to improve overall performance. It takes advantage of the particular effectiveness of each training method, while at the same time attempting to neglect the shortcomings of that method by combining it with other methods that address its weaknesses. With respect to employee-employer relationship, cross training refers to the training of one employee to do another's work.

Heart rate	Heart rate is the number of heartbeats per unit of time - typically expressed as beats per minute (BPM) - which can vary as the body's need for oxygen changes, such as during exercise or sleep. The measurement of Heart rate is used by medical professionals to assist in the diagnosis and tracking of medical conditions. It is also used by individuals, such as athletes, who are interested in monitoring their Heart rate to gain maximum efficiency from their training.
Exercise intensity	Exercise intensity refers to how much work is being done when exercising. The intensity has an effect on what fuel the body uses and what kind of adaptations the body makes after exercise (i.e., the training effect). Fuel used The body uses different amounts of fuels (carbohydrate or fat) depending on the intensity and heart rate.
Water activity	Water activity or a_w was developed to account for the intensity with which water associates with various non-aqueous constituents. Simply stated, it is a measure of the energy status of the water in a system. It is defined as the vapor pressure of a liquid divided by that of pure water at the same temperature; therefore, pure distilled water has a water activity of exactly one.
Health care	Health care , refers to the treatment and management of illness, and the preservation of health through services offered by the medical, dental, complementary and alternative medicine, pharmaceutical, clinical laboratory sciences , nursing, and allied health professions. Health care embraces all the goods and services designed to promote health, including 'preventive, curative and palliative interventions, whether directed to individuals or to populations'. Before the term Health care became popular, English-speakers referred to medicine or to the health sector and spoke of the treatment and prevention of illness and disease.
Stretching	Stretching is a form of physical exercise in which a specific skeletal muscle (or muscle group) is deliberately elongated, often by abduction from the torso, in order to improve the muscle's felt elasticity and reaffirm comfortable muscle tone. The result is a feeling of increased muscle control, flexibility and range of motion. Stretching is also used therapeutically to alleviate cramps.
Diaphragmatic breathing	Diaphragmatic breathing, abdominal breathing, belly breathing, deep breathing or costal breathing is the act of breathing deep into one's lungs by flexing one's diaphragm rather than breathing shallowly by flexing one's rib cage. This deep breathing is marked by expansion of the stomach (abdomen) rather than the chest when breathing. It is generally considered a healthier and fuller way to ingest oxygen, and is often used as a therapy for hyperventilation and anxiety disorders.

Chapter 12. Exercise,

Diabetes mellitus	Diabetes mellitus strikes 1 in 400 cats and a similar number of dogs, though recent veterinary studies note that it is becoming more common lately in cats. Symptoms in dogs and cats are similar to those in humans. Generally, most dogs and about 5-20% of cats experience type-1 (insulin-dependent) diabetes, rather than the type-2 that's now becoming common in obese humans.
Rhythm	Rhythm is the variation of the length and accentuation of a series of sounds or other events. The study of Rhythm, stress, and pitch in speech is called prosody; it is a topic in linguistics. Narmour (1980, p. 147-53) describes three categories of prosodic rules which create Rhythmic successions which are additive (same duration repeated), cumulative (short-long), or countercumulative (long-short).
Data collection	Data collection is a term used to describe a process of preparing and collecting data - for example as part of a process improvement or similar project. The purpose of Data collection is to obtain information to keep on record, to make decisions about important issues, to pass information on to others. Primarily, data is collected to provide information regarding a specific topic. Data collection usually takes place early on in an improvement project, and is often formalised through a Data collection plan which often contains the following activity. · Pre collection activity - Agree goals, target data, definitions, methods· Collection - Data collection· Present Findings - usually involves some form of sorting analysis and/or presentation.

Chapter 12. Exercise,

1. _____ or _____s refers to the class of diseases that involve the heart or blood vessels (arteries and veins). While the term technically refers to any disease that affects the cardiovascular system (as used in MeSH), it is usually used to refer to those related to atherosclerosis (arterial disease). These conditions have similar causes, mechanisms, and treatments.

   a. Bacteriophage
   b. Fascia
   c. Cardiovascular disease
   d. Baroreflex

2. _____ is the variation of the length and accentuation of a series of sounds or other events.

   The study of _____, stress, and pitch in speech is called prosody; it is a topic in linguistics. Narmour (1980, p. 147-53) describes three categories of prosodic rules which create Rhythmic successions which are additive (same duration repeated), cumulative (short-long), or countercumulative (long-short).

   a. Bacteriophage
   b. Premium
   c. Rhythm
   d. Binocular vision

3. _____ is cancer originating from breast tissue, most commonly from the inner lining of milk ducts or the lobules that supply the ducts with milk. Cancers originating from ducts are known as ductal carcinomas; those originating from lobules are known as lobular carcinomas.

   The size, stage, rate of growth, and other characteristics of the tumor determine the kinds of treatment.

   a. Breast Cancer Action
   b. Breast cancer
   c. Breast Cancer Care
   d. Breast Cancer Research and Treatment

4. _____ is a chronic, systemic inflammatory disorder that may affect many tissues and organs, but principally attacks the joints producing an inflammatory synovitis that often progresses to destruction of the articular cartilage and ankylosis of the joints. _____ can also produce diffuse inflammation in the lungs, pericardium, pleura, and sclera, and also nodular lesions, most common in subcutaneous tissue under the skin. Although the cause of _____ is unknown, autoimmunity plays a pivotal role in its chronicity and progression.

   a. Rheumatoid arthritis
   b. Scleredema adultorum
   c. Scleredema of Buschke
   d. Systemic lupus erythematosus

5. . A _____ is a research methodology common in social science. It is based on an in-depth investigation of a single individual, group, or event to explore causation in order to find underlying principles.

a. Bacteriophage

b. Case study

c. Herbal tobacco alternatives

d. Canadian Blood Services

1. c
2. c
3. b
4. a
5. b

You can take the complete Chapter Practice Test

for Chapter 12. Exercise,
on all key terms, persons, places, and concepts.

Online 99 Cents

http://www.epub1625.32.20273.12.cram101.com/

Use www.Cram101.com for all your study needs

including Cram101's online interactive problem solving labs in

chemistry, statistics, mathematics, and more.

	Problem solving
	Eustress
	Musculoskeletal system
	Nervous system
	Case study
	Health care
	Heart rate
	Resistance training
	Respiratory rate
	Exercise intensity
	Nutrition
	Sleep hygiene
	Postpartum depression
	Empathy

CHAPTER HIGHLIGHTS & NOTES: KEY TERMS, PEOPLE, PLACES, CONCEPTS

Problem solving	Problem solving is a mental process and is part of the larger problem process that includes problem finding and problem shaping.

Considered the most complex of all intellectual functions, Problem solving has been defined as higher-order cognitive process that requires the modulation and control of more routine or fundamental skills. Problem solving occurs when an organism or an artificial intelligence system needs to move from a given state to a desired goal state.

Eustress

Eustress is a term coined by endocrinologist Hans Selye which is defined in the model of Richard Lazarus (1974) as stress that is healthy, or gives one a feeling of fulfillment or other positive feelings. Eustress is a process of exploring potential gains.

Etymology

The word eustress consists of two parts.

Musculoskeletal system

A Musculoskeletal system is an organ system that gives animals (including humans) the ability to move using the muscular and skeletal systems. The Musculoskeletal system provides form, stability, and movement to the body.

It is made up of the body's bones (the skeleton), muscles, cartilage, tendons, ligaments, joints, and other connective tissue (the tissue that supports and binds tissues and organs together).

Nervous system

The Nervous system is an organ system containing a network of specialized cells called neurons that coordinate the actions of an animal and transmit signals between different parts of its body. In most animals the Nervous system consists of two parts, central and peripheral. The central Nervous system contains the brain and spinal cord.

Case study

A Case study is a research methodology common in social science. It is based on an in-depth investigation of a single individual, group, or event to explore causation in order to find underlying principles.

Health care

Health care , refers to the treatment and management of illness, and the preservation of health through services offered by the medical, dental, complementary and alternative medicine, pharmaceutical, clinical laboratory sciences , nursing, and allied health professions. Health care embraces all the goods and services designed to promote health, including 'preventive, curative and palliative interventions, whether directed to individuals or to populations'.

Before the term Health care became popular, English-speakers referred to medicine or to the health sector and spoke of the treatment and prevention of illness and disease.

Heart rate

Heart rate is the number of heartbeats per unit of time - typically expressed as beats per minute (BPM) - which can vary as the body's need for oxygen changes, such as during exercise or sleep.

Chapter 13. Stress Management,

The measurement of Heart rate is used by medical professionals to assist in the diagnosis and tracking of medical conditions. It is also used by individuals, such as athletes, who are interested in monitoring their Heart rate to gain maximum efficiency from their training.

| Resistance training | Resistance training has two different meanings. |

| Respiratory rate | Respiratory rate (aka respiration rate, pulmonary ventilation rate or ventilation rate) is the number of breaths a living being, such as a human, takes within a certain amount of time (frequently given in breaths per minute).

There is only limited research on monitoring Respiratory rate, and these studies have focused on such issues as the inaccuracy of Respiratory rate measurement and Respiratory rate as a marker for respiratory dysfunction.

The human respiration rate is usually measured when a person is at rest and simply involves counting the number of breaths for one minute by counting how many times the chest rises. |

| Exercise intensity | Exercise intensity refers to how much work is being done when exercising. The intensity has an effect on what fuel the body uses and what kind of adaptations the body makes after exercise (i.e., the training effect).

Fuel used

The body uses different amounts of fuels (carbohydrate or fat) depending on the intensity and heart rate. |

| Nutrition | Nutrition is the provision, to cells and organisms, of the materials necessary (in the form of food) to support life. Many common health problems can be prevented or alleviated with a healthy diet.

The diet of an organism is what it eats, and is largely determined by the perceived palatability of foods. |

| Sleep hygiene | Sleep hygiene can be defined as the controlling of 'all behavioural and environmental factors that precede sleep and may interfere with sleep.' It is the practice of following guidelines in an attempt to ensure more restful, effective sleep which can promote daytime alertness and help treat or avoid certain kinds of sleep disorders. Trouble sleeping and daytime sleepiness can be indications of poor Sleep hygiene. The International Classification of Sleep Disorders-Revised (ICSD-R) states on page 75: 'The importance of assessing the contribution of inadequate Sleep hygiene in maintaining a preexisting sleep disturbance cannot be overemphasized.' |

Chapter 13. Stress Management,

Postpartum depression	Postpartum depression (PPostpartum depression) is a form of clinical depression which can affect women, and less frequently men, after childbirth. Studies report prevalence rates among women from 5% to 25%, but methodological differences among the studies make the actual prevalence rate unclear. Postpartum depression occurs in women after they have carried a child, usually in the first few months.
Empathy	Empathy is the capacity to recognize and, to some extent, share feelings (such as sadness or happiness) that are being experienced by another semi-sentient being. Someone may need to have a certain amount of empathy before they are able to feel compassion. Etymology The English word is derived from the Greek word ?μπ?θεια (empatheia), 'physical affection, passion, partiality' which comes from ?v (en), 'in, at' + π?θος (pathos), 'passion' or 'suffering'.

1. A _____ is an organ system that gives animals (including humans) the ability to move using the muscular and skeletal systems. The _____ provides form, stability, and movement to the body.

   It is made up of the body's bones (the skeleton), muscles, cartilage, tendons, ligaments, joints, and other connective tissue (the tissue that supports and binds tissues and organs together).

   a. Plantarflexion
   b. Fascia
   c. Musculoskeletal system
   d. Bacteriophage

2. A _____ is a research methodology common in social science. It is based on an in-depth investigation of a single individual, group, or event to explore causation in order to find underlying principles.

   a. Bacteriophage
   b. Biological system
   c. Case study
   d. Benign prostatic hyperplasia

3. . _____ (aka respiration rate, pulmonary ventilation rate or ventilation rate) is the number of breaths a living being, such as a human, takes within a certain amount of time (frequently given in breaths per minute).

   There is only limited research on monitoring _____, and these studies have focused on such issues as the inaccuracy of _____ measurement and _____ as a marker for respiratory dysfunction.

Chapter 13. Stress Management,

The human respiration rate is usually measured when a person is at rest and simply involves counting the number of breaths for one minute by counting how many times the chest rises.

    a. Pallor
    b. Papilledema
    c. Petechia
    d. Respiratory rate

4. The _____ is an organ system containing a network of specialized cells called neurons that coordinate the actions of an animal and transmit signals between different parts of its body. In most animals the _____ consists of two parts, central and peripheral. The central _____ contains the brain and spinal cord.

    a. Metric system
    b. Nervous system
    c. Bacteriophage
    d. Baroreflex

5. _____ (PPostpartum depression) is a form of clinical depression which can affect women, and less frequently men, after childbirth. Studies report prevalence rates among women from 5% to 25%, but methodological differences among the studies make the actual prevalence rate unclear. _____ occurs in women after they have carried a child, usually in the first few months.

    a. Seasonal affective disorder
    b. Bacteriophage
    c. Baroreflex
    d. Postpartum depression

ANSWER KEY
Chapter 13. Stress Management,

1. c
2. c
3. d
4. b
5. d

You can take the complete Chapter Practice Test

for Chapter 13. Stress Management,
on all key terms, persons, places, and concepts.

Online 99 Cents

http://www.epub1625.32.20273.13.cram101.com/

Use www.Cram101.com for all your study needs

including Cram101's online interactive problem solving labs in

chemistry, statistics, mathematics, and more.

Chapter 14. Holistic Health Strategies,

Holistic health

Allopathic medicine

Health promotion

Bodywork

Acupuncture

Moxibustion

Acupressure

Reflexology

Shiatsu

Substance abuse

Therapeutic touch

Polarity therapy

Meditation

Mindfulness

Craniosacral therapy

CHAPTER HIGHLIGHTS & NOTES: KEY TERMS, PEOPLE, PLACES, CONCEPTS

Holistic health	Holistic health is a concept in medical practice upholding that all aspects of people's needs, psychological, physical and social, should be taken into account and seen as a whole. As defined above, the holistic view on treatment is widely accepted in medicine. A different definition, claiming that disease is a result of physical, emotional, spiritual, social and environmental imbalance, is used in alternative medicine.
Allopathic medicine	Allopathic medicine and allopathy are terms coined by Samuel Hahnemann, the founder of homeopathy. It meant 'other than the disease' and it was intended, among other things, to point out how traditional doctors used methods that had nothing to do with the symptoms created by the disease and which, in Hahnemann's view, meant that these methods were harmful to the patients.

Originally intended as a characterization of standard medicine in the early 19th century, these terms were rejected by mainstream physicians and quickly acquired negative overtones. |
| Health promotion | Health promotion has been defined by the World Health Organization's 2005 Bangkok Charter for Health promotion in a Globalized World as 'the process of enabling people to increase control over their health and its determinants, and thereby improve their health'. The primary means of Health promotion occur through developing healthy public policy that addresses the prerequisities of health such as income, housing, food security, employment, and quality working conditions. There is a tendency among public health officials and governments -- and this is especially the case in liberal nations such as Canada and the USA -- to reduce Health promotion to health education and social marketing focused on changing behavioral risk factors. |
| Bodywork | In automotive engineering, the Bodywork of an automobile is the structure which protects:

· The occupants · Any other payload · The mechanical components.

In vehicles with a separate frame or chassis, the term Bodywork is normally applied to only the non-structural panels, including doors and other movable panels, but it may also be used more generally to include the structural components which support the mechanical components.

There are three main types of automotive Bodywork:

· The first automobiles were designs adapted in large part from horse-drawn carriages, and had body-on-frame construction with a wooden frame and wooden or metal body panels. |
| Acupuncture | Acupuncture is the procedure of inserting and manipulating needles into various points on the body to relieve pain or for therapeutic purposes. The earliest written record of Acupuncture is the Chinese text Shiji with elaboration of its history in the second century BCE medical text Huangdi Neijing . |

Chapter 14. Holistic Health Strategies,

Moxibustion	Moxibustion is a traditional Chinese medicine therapy using moxa, or mugwort herb. It plays an important role in the traditional medical systems of China, Japan, Korea, Vietnam, Tibet, and Mongolia. Suppliers usually age the mugwort and grind it up to a fluff; practitioners burn the fluff or process it further into a stick that resembles a cigar.
Acupressure	Acupressure is a complementary medicine technique derived from acupuncture. In Acupressure physical pressure is applied to acupuncture points by the hand, elbow, or with various devices. Traditional Chinese medicine's acupuncture theory predates use of the scientific method, and has received various criticisms based on scientific thinking.
Reflexology	Reflexology (zone therapy) is an alternative medicine method involving the practice of massaging , or sometimes the hands and ears, with the goal of encouraging a beneficial effect on other parts of the body, or to improve general health. The Reflexology Association of Canada defines Reflexology as: A natural healing art based on the principle that there are reflexes in the feet, hands and ears and their referral areas within zone related areas, which correspond to every part, gland and organ of the body. Through application of pressure on these reflexes without the use of tools, crèmes or lotions, the feet being the primary area of application, Reflexology relieves tension, improves circulation and helps promote the natural function of the related areas of the body.
Shiatsu	Shiatsu is a traditional hands-on therapy originating in Japan. There are two main Shiatsu schools; one based on western anatomical and physiological theory and the other based on Traditional Chinese Medicine . Shiatsu is regulated as a licensed medical therapy in Japan by the Ministry of Health and Welfare, and elsewhere by various governing bodies set up by Shiatsu practitioners.
Substance abuse	Substance abuse also known as drug abuse, refers to a maladaptive pattern of use of a substance that is not considered dependent. The term 'drug abuse' does not exclude dependency, but is otherwise used in a similar manner in nonmedical contexts. The terms have a huge range of definitions related to taking a psychoactive drug or performance enhancing drug for a non-therapeutic or non-medical effect.
Therapeutic touch	Therapeutic touch (commonly shortened to),) or Distance Healing, is an energy therapy claimed to promote healing and reduce pain and anxiety. Practitioners of Therapeutic touch claim that by placing their hands on, or near, a patient, they are able to detect and manipulate the patient's putative energy field. Although there are currently (September 2009) 259 articles concerning Therapeutic touch on PubMed the quality of controlled research and tests is variable.
Polarity therapy	· Energy (esotericism) · Electromagnetic therapy · Polarity therapy · Reiki

Meditation	Meditation is a mental discipline by which one attempts to get beyond the reflexive, 'thinking' mind into a deeper state of relaxation or awareness. Meditation often involves turning attention to a single point of reference. It is a component of many religions, and has been practiced since antiquity.
Mindfulness	Mindfulness is calm awareness of one's body functions, feelings, content of consciousness, or consciousness itself. Mindfulness plays a central role in the teaching of the Buddha where it is affirmed that 'correct' or 'right' Mindfulness is the critical factor in the path to liberation and subsequent enlightenment. It is the seventh element of the Noble Eightfold Path, the practice of which supports analysis resulting in the development of wisdom .
Craniosacral therapy	Craniosacral therapy (, cranial osteopathy, also spelled CranioSacral bodywork or therapy) is a method of Complementary and alternative medicine used by physical therapists, occupational therapists, massage therapists, naturopaths, chiropractors and osteopaths. A Craniosacral therapy session involves the therapist placing their hands on the patient, which they say allows them to tune into what they call the craniosacral system. By gently working with the spine, the skull and its cranial sutures, diaphragms, and fascia, the restrictions of nerve passages are said to be eased, the movement of cerebrospinal fluid through the spinal cord can be optimized, and misaligned bones are said to be restored to their proper position.

CHAPTER QUIZ: KEY TERMS, PEOPLE, PLACES, CONCEPTS

1. _____ is a concept in medical practice upholding that all aspects of people's needs, psychological, physical and social, should be taken into account and seen as a whole. As defined above, the holistic view on treatment is widely accepted in medicine. A different definition, claiming that disease is a result of physical, emotional, spiritual, social and environmental imbalance, is used in alternative medicine.

   a. Bacteriophage
   b. Baroreflex
   c. Holistic health
   d. Benzathine benzylpenicillin

2. . _____ and allopathy are terms coined by Samuel Hahnemann, the founder of homeopathy. It meant 'other than the disease' and it was intended, among other things, to point out how traditional doctors used methods that had nothing to do with the symptoms created by the disease and which, in Hahnemann's view, meant that these methods were harmful to the patients.

   Originally intended as a characterization of standard medicine in the early 19th century, these terms were rejected by mainstream physicians and quickly acquired negative overtones.

   a. Allopathic medicine

Chapter 14. Holistic Health Strategies,

    b. Epicardial

    c. Auditory agnosia

    d. Afferent

3. _____ has been defined by the World Health Organization's 2005 Bangkok Charter for _____ in a Globalized World as 'the process of enabling people to increase control over their health and its determinants, and thereby improve their health'. The primary means of _____ occur through developing healthy public policy that addresses the prerequisities of health such as income, housing, food security, employment, and quality working conditions. There is a tendency among public health officials and governments -- and this is especially the case in liberal nations such as Canada and the USA -- to reduce _____ to health education and social marketing focused on changing behavioral risk factors.

    a. Bacteriophage

    b. Health promotion

    c. Auditory agnosia

    d. Afferent

4. _____ (zone therapy) is an alternative medicine method involving the practice of massaging , or sometimes the hands and ears, with the goal of encouraging a beneficial effect on other parts of the body, or to improve general health.

The _____ Association of Canada defines _____ as: A natural healing art based on the principle that there are reflexes in the feet, hands and ears and their referral areas within zone related areas, which correspond to every part, gland and organ of the body. Through application of pressure on these reflexes without the use of tools, crèmes or lotions, the feet being the primary area of application, _____ relieves tension, improves circulation and helps promote the natural function of the related areas of the body.

    a. Bacteriophage

    b. Effleurage

    c. Reflexology

    d. Acupoint therapy

5. . In automotive engineering, the _____ of an automobile is the structure which protects:

· The occupants · Any other payload · The mechanical components.

In vehicles with a separate frame or chassis, the term _____ is normally applied to only the non-structural panels, including doors and other movable panels, but it may also be used more generally to include the structural components which support the mechanical components.

There are three main types of automotive _____:

· The first automobiles were designs adapted in large part from horse-drawn carriages, and had body-on-frame construction with a wooden frame and wooden or metal body panels.

    a. Bacteriophage

b. Epicardial

c. Auditory agnosia

d. Bodywork

1. c
2. a
3. b
4. c
5. d

You can take the complete Chapter Practice Test

for Chapter 14. Holistic Health Strategies,
on all key terms, persons, places, and concepts.

Online 99 Cents

http://www.epub1625.32.20273.14.cram101.com/

Use www.Cram101.com for all your study needs

including Cram101's online interactive problem solving labs in

chemistry, statistics, mathematics, and more.

	Growth chart
	Denver Developmental Screening Test
	Cognitive development
	Cardiovascular disease

Growth chart	A Growth chart is used by pediatricians and other health care providers to follow a child's growth over time. Growth charts have been constructed by observing the growth of large numbers of normal children over time. The height, weight, and head circumference of a child can be compared to the expected parameters of children of the same age and sex to determine whether the child is growing appropriately.
Denver Developmental Screening Test	The Denver Developmental Screening Test , commonly known as the Denver Scale, is a test for screening cognitive and behavioural problems in preschool children. It was developed by William K. Frankenburg and first introduced by him and J.B. Dobbs in 1967. The test is currently marketed by Denver Developmental Materials, Inc., in Denver, Colorado, hence the name.
Cognitive development	Cognitive development is a field of study in neuroscience and psychology focusing on a child's development in terms of information processing, conceptual resources, perceptual skill, language learning, and other aspects of brain development and cognitive psychology. A large portion of research has gone into understanding how a child conceptualizes the world. Jean Piaget was a major force in the founding of this field, forming his 'theory of Cognitive development'.
Cardiovascular disease	Cardiovascular disease or Cardiovascular diseases refers to the class of diseases that involve the heart or blood vessels (arteries and veins). While the term technically refers to any disease that affects the cardiovascular system (as used in MeSH), it is usually used to refer to those related to atherosclerosis (arterial disease). These conditions have similar causes, mechanisms, and treatments.

Chapter 15. Overview of Growth and Development Framework,

1. A _____ is used by pediatricians and other health care providers to follow a child's growth over time. _____s have been constructed by observing the growth of large numbers of normal children over time. The height, weight, and head circumference of a child can be compared to the expected parameters of children of the same age and sex to determine whether the child is growing appropriately.

   a. Tricuspid atresia
   b. Growth chart
   c. Baroreflex
   d. Benign prostatic hyperplasia

2. _____ is a field of study in neuroscience and psychology focusing on a child's development in terms of information processing, conceptual resources, perceptual skill, language learning, and other aspects of brain development and cognitive psychology. A large portion of research has gone into understanding how a child conceptualizes the world. Jean Piaget was a major force in the founding of this field, forming his 'theory of _____'.

   a. Bacteriophage
   b. Cognitive development
   c. Benign prostatic hyperplasia
   d. Benzathine benzylpenicillin

3. _____ or _____s refers to the class of diseases that involve the heart or blood vessels (arteries and veins). While the term technically refers to any disease that affects the cardiovascular system (as used in MeSH), it is usually used to refer to those related to atherosclerosis (arterial disease). These conditions have similar causes, mechanisms, and treatments.

   a. Bacteriophage
   b. Baroreflex
   c. Benign prostatic hyperplasia
   d. Cardiovascular disease

4. The _____ , commonly known as the Denver Scale, is a test for screening cognitive and behavioural problems in preschool children. It was developed by William K. Frankenburg and first introduced by him and J.B. Dobbs in 1967. The test is currently marketed by Denver Developmental Materials, Inc., in Denver, Colorado, hence the name.

   a. Tricuspid atresia
   b. Denver Developmental Screening Test
   c. Baroreflex
   d. Benign prostatic hyperplasia

1. b
2. b
3. d
4. b

You can take the complete Chapter Practice Test

for Chapter 15. Overview of Growth and Development Framework,
on all key terms, persons, places, and concepts.

Online 99 Cents

http://www.epub1625.32.20273.15.cram101.com/

Use www.Cram101.com for all your study needs

including Cram101's online interactive problem solving labs in

chemistry, statistics, mathematics, and more.

Chapter 16. The Prenatal Period,

CHAPTER OUTLINE: KEY TERMS, PEOPLE, PLACES, CONCEPTS

Prenatal care

Chorionic villi

Cardiovascular disease

Health care

Life expectancy

Cardiovascular system

Integumentary system

Linea nigra

Musculoskeletal system

Reproductive health

Respiratory system

Striae gravidarum

Pregnancy

Hepatitis B

Health education

Weight gain

Case study

Health promotion

Apgar score

Visit Cram101.com for full Practice Exams

Chapter 16. The Prenatal Period,

_____ | Heart rate

_____ | Meconium

_____ | Exercise intensity

_____ | Cleft palate

_____ | Amniocentesis

_____ | Down syndrome

_____ | Trisomy

_____ | Nutrition

_____ | Health effect

_____ | Quickening

_____ | Urinary system

_____ | Polyhydramnios

_____ | Toxoplasmosis

_____ | Syphilis

_____ | Cytomegalovirus

_____ | Candida albicans

_____ | Herpes simplex

_____ | Blood type

_____ | Prescription drug

	Fetal alcohol syndrome
	Amniotic fluid
	Data collection
	Smoking cessation
	Home birth

CHAPTER HIGHLIGHTS & NOTES: KEY TERMS, PEOPLE, PLACES, CONCEPTS

Prenatal care	Prenatal care refers to the medical and nursing care recommended for women before and during pregnancy. The aim of good Prenatal care is to detect any potential problems early, to prevent them if possible (through recommendations on adequate nutrition, exercise, vitamin intake etc), and to direct the woman to appropriate specialists, hospitals, etc. if necessary.
Chorionic villi	Chorionic villi are villi that sprout from the chorion in order to give a maximum area of contact with the maternal blood. Embryonic blood is carried to the villi by the branches of the umbilical arteries, and after circulating through the capillaries of the villi, is returned to the embryo by the umbilical veins. Thus, the villi are part of the border between maternal and fetal blood during pregnancy.
Cardiovascular disease	Cardiovascular disease or Cardiovascular diseases refers to the class of diseases that involve the heart or blood vessels (arteries and veins). While the term technically refers to any disease that affects the cardiovascular system (as used in MeSH), it is usually used to refer to those related to atherosclerosis (arterial disease). These conditions have similar causes, mechanisms, and treatments.
Health care	Health care , refers to the treatment and management of illness, and the preservation of health through services offered by the medical, dental, complementary and alternative medicine, pharmaceutical, clinical laboratory sciences , nursing, and allied health professions.

Chapter 16. The Prenatal Period,

Health care embraces all the goods and services designed to promote health, including 'preventive, curative and palliative interventions, whether directed to individuals or to populations'.

Before the term Health care became popular, English-speakers referred to medicine or to the health sector and spoke of the treatment and prevention of illness and disease.

Life expectancy	Life expectancy is the average number of years of life remaining at a given age. The term is most often used in the human context, but used also in plant or animal ecology and the calculation is based on the analysis of life tables (also known as actuarial tables). The term may also be used in the context of manufactured objects although the related term shelf life is used for consumer products and the term mean time to breakdown (MTTB) is used in engineering literature.
Cardiovascular system	The circulatory system is an organ system that passes nutrients (such as amino acids and electrolytes), gases, hormones, blood cells, etc. to and from cells in the body to help fight diseases and help stabilize body temperature and pH to maintain homeostasis. This system may be seen strictly as a blood distribution network, but some consider the circulatory system as composed of the Cardiovascular system, which distributes blood, and the lymphatic system, which distributes lymph.
Integumentary system	'Integument' redirects here; in botany, an integument is an outer membrane of an ovule, which later develops into a seed coat.
	The Integumentary system is the organ system that protects the body from damage, comprising the skin and its appendages . The Integumentary system has a variety of functions; it may serve to waterproof, cushion and protect the deeper tissues, excrete wastes, regulate temperature and is the attachment site for sensory receptors to detect pain, sensation, pressure and temperature.
Linea nigra	Linea nigra is a dark vertical line that appears on the abdomen during about three quarters of all pregnancies. The brownish streak is usually about a centimeter in width. The line runs vertically along the midline of the abdomen from the pubis to the xiphoid process.
Musculoskeletal system	A Musculoskeletal system is an organ system that gives animals (including humans) the ability to move using the muscular and skeletal systems. The Musculoskeletal system provides form, stability, and movement to the body.
	It is made up of the body's bones (the skeleton), muscles, cartilage, tendons, ligaments, joints, and other connective tissue (the tissue that supports and binds tissues and organs together).

Reproductive health	Within the framework of WHO's definition of health as a state of complete physical, mental and social well-being, and not merely the absence of disease or infirmity, reproductive health, addresses the reproductive processes, functions and system at all stages of life. Reproductive health, therefore, implies that people are able to have a responsible, satisfying and safer sex life and that they have the capability to reproduce and the freedom to decide if, when and how often to do so. Implicit in this are the right of men and women to be informed of and to have access to safe, effective, affordable and acceptable methods of birth control of their choice; and the right of access to appropriate health care services that will enable women to go safely through pregnancy and childbirth and provide couples with the best chance of having a healthy infant.
Respiratory system	The respiratory system's function is to allow gas exchange to all parts of the body. The space between the alveoli and the capillaries, the anatomy or structure of the exchange system, and the precise physiological uses of the exchanged gases vary depending on the organism. In humans and other mammals, for example, the anatomical features of the respiratory system include airways, lungs, and the respiratory muscles.
Striae gravidarum	Striae gravidarum are a cutaneous condition characterized by stretch marks on the abdomen following pregnancy. .
Pregnancy	Pregnancy is the carrying of one or more offspring, known as a fetus or embryo, inside the womb of a female. In a pregnancy, there can be multiple gestations, as in the case of twins or triplets. Human pregnancy is the most studied of all mammalian pregnancies.
Hepatitis B	Hepatitis B is an infectious illness caused by hepatitis B virus (HBV) which infects the liver of hominoidea, including humans, and causes an inflammation called hepatitis. Originally known as 'serum hepatitis', the disease has caused epidemics in parts of Asia and Africa, and it is endemic in China. About a third of the world's population, more than 2 billion people, have been infected with the hepatitis B virus.
Health education	Health education is the profession of educating people about health. Areas within this profession encompass environmental health, physical health, social health, emotional health, intellectual health, and spiritual health. It can be defined as the principle by which individuals and groups of people learn to behave in a manner conducive to the promotion, maintenance, or restoration of health.
Weight gain	Weight gain is an increase in body weight. This can be either an increase in muscle mass, fat deposits, or excess fluids such as water. Description

Chapter 16. The Prenatal Period,

Case study	A Case study is a research methodology common in social science. It is based on an in-depth investigation of a single individual, group, or event to explore causation in order to find underlying principles.
Health promotion	Health promotion has been defined by the World Health Organization's 2005 Bangkok Charter for Health promotion in a Globalized World as 'the process of enabling people to increase control over their health and its determinants, and thereby improve their health'. The primary means of Health promotion occur through developing healthy public policy that addresses the prerequisities of health such as income, housing, food security, employment, and quality working conditions. There is a tendency among public health officials and governments -- and this is especially the case in liberal nations such as Canada and the USA -- to reduce Health promotion to health education and social marketing focused on changing behavioral risk factors.
Apgar score	The Apgar score was devised in 1952 by Dr. Virginia Apgar as a simple and repeatable method to quickly and summarily assess the health of newborn children immediately after childbirth. Apgar was an anesthesiologist who developed the score in order to ascertain the effects of obstetric anesthesia on babies. The Apgar score is determined by evaluating the newborn baby on five simple criteria on a scale from zero to two, then summing up the five values thus obtained.
Heart rate	Heart rate is the number of heartbeats per unit of time - typically expressed as beats per minute (BPM) - which can vary as the body's need for oxygen changes, such as during exercise or sleep. The measurement of Heart rate is used by medical professionals to assist in the diagnosis and tracking of medical conditions. It is also used by individuals, such as athletes, who are interested in monitoring their Heart rate to gain maximum efficiency from their training.
Meconium	Meconium is the earliest stools of an infant. Unlike later feces, Meconium is composed of materials ingested during the time the infant spends in the uterus: intestinal epithelial cells, lanugo, mucus, amniotic fluid, bile, and water. Meconium is almost sterile, unlike later feces, is viscous and sticky like tar, and has no odor.
Exercise intensity	Exercise intensity refers to how much work is being done when exercising. The intensity has an effect on what fuel the body uses and what kind of adaptations the body makes after exercise (i.e., the training effect). Fuel used The body uses different amounts of fuels (carbohydrate or fat) depending on the intensity and heart rate.

Cleft palate	Cleft lip (cheiloschisis) and Cleft palate (colloquially known as harelip), which can also occur together as cleft lip and palate, are variations of a type of clefting congenital deformity caused by abnormal facial development during gestation. A cleft is a fissure or opening--a gap. It is the non-fusion of the body's natural structures that form before birth.
Amniocentesis	Amniocentesis is a medical procedure used in prenatal diagnosis of chromosomal abnormalities and fetal infections , in which a small amount of amniotic fluid, which contains fetal tissues, is extracted from the amnion or amniotic sac surrounding a developing fetus, and the fetal DNA is examined for genetic abnormalities.
	Before the start of the procedure, a local anesthetic can be given to the mother in order to relieve the pain felt during the insertion of the needle used to withdraw the fluid. After the local is in effect, a needle is usually inserted through the mother's abdominal wall, then through the wall of the uterus, and finally into the amniotic sac.
Down syndrome	Down syndrome, trisomy 21, is a chromosomal condition caused by the presence of all or part of an extra 21st chromosome. It is named after John Langdon Down, the British physician who described the syndrome in 1866. The condition was identified as a chromosome 21 trisomy by Jérôme Lejeune in 1959. Down syndrome in a fetus can be identified with amniocentesis (with risks of fetal injury and/or miscarriage) during pregnancy, or in a baby at birth.
	Down syndrome is a chromosomal condition characterized by the presence of an extra copy of genetic material on the 21st chromosome, either in whole (trisomy 21) or part (such as due to translocations).
Trisomy	A Trisomy is a genetic abnormality in which there are three copies, instead of the normal two, of a particular chromosome. A Trisomy is a type of aneuploidy (an abnormal number of chromosomes).
	Most organisms that reproduce sexually have pairs of chromosomes in each cell, with one chromosome inherited from each parent.
Nutrition	Nutrition is the provision, to cells and organisms, of the materials necessary (in the form of food) to support life. Many common health problems can be prevented or alleviated with a healthy diet.
	The diet of an organism is what it eats, and is largely determined by the perceived palatability of foods.
Health effect	Health effects are changes in health resulting from exposure to a source. Health effects are an important consideration in many areas, such as hygiene, pollution studies, workplace safety, nutrition and health sciences in general.

Chapter 16. The Prenatal Period,

Quickening	In pregnancy terms, the moment of Quickening refers to the initial motion of the fetus in the uterus as it is perceived or felt by the pregnant woman. According to the Oxford English Dictionary, to 'quicken' means 'to reach the stage of pregnancy at which the child shows signs of life.' In the twentieth century, ultrasound technology made it possible to see that a fetus is in motion even if the pregnant woman does not yet feel it. This technological development made the concept of 'Quickening' a bit more complex.
Urinary system	The Urinary system is the organ system that produces, stores, and eliminates urine. In humans it includes two kidneys, two ureters, the bladder, the urethra, and the penis in males. The analogous organ in invertebrates is the nephridium.
Polyhydramnios	Polyhydramnios (polyhydramnion, hydramnios) is a medical condition describing an excess of amniotic fluid in the amniotic sac. It is seen in 0.5 to 5% of pregnancies. It is typically diagnosed when the amniotic fluid exceeds 2000 mL. The opposite to Polyhydramnios is oligohydramnios, a deficiency in amniotic fluid.
Toxoplasmosis	Toxoplasmosis is a parasitic disease caused by the protozoan Toxoplasma gondii. The parasite infects most genera of warm-blooded animals, including humans, but the primary host is the felid (cat) family. Animals are infected by eating infected meat, by ingestion of feces of a cat that has itself recently been infected, or by transmission from mother to fetus.
Syphilis	Syphilis is a sexually transmitted disease caused by the spirochetal bacteria Treponema pallidum subspecies pallidum. The primary route of transmission of syphilis is through sexual contact however it may also be transmitted from mother to fetus during pregnancy or at birth resulting in congenital syphilis. The signs and symptoms of syphilis vary depending on which of the four stages it presents in (primary, secondary, latent, and tertiary).
Cytomegalovirus	Cytomegalovirus is a herpes viral genus of the Herpesviruses group: in humans it is commonly known as HCMV or Human Herpesvirus 5 (HHV-5). CMV belongs to the Betaherpesvirinae subfamily of Herpesviridae, which also includes Roseolovirus. Other herpesviruses fall into the subfamilies of Alphaherpesvirinae (including HSV 1 and 2 and varicella) or Gammaherpesvirinae (including Epstein-Barr virus).
Candida albicans	Candida albicans is a diploid fungus (a form of yeast) and a causal agent of opportunistic oral and genital infections in humans. Systemic fungal infections (fungemias) have emerged as important causes of morbidity and mortality in immunocompromised patients (e.g., AIDS, cancer chemotherapy, organ or bone marrow transplantation).

Herpes simplex	Herpes simplex is a viral disease caused by both herpes simplex virus type 1 (HSV-1) and type 2 (HSV-2). Infection with the herpes virus is categorized into one of several distinct disorders based on the site of infection. Oral herpes, the visible symptoms of which are colloquially called cold sores or fever blisters, infects the face and mouth.
Blood type	A Blood type is a classification of blood based on the presence or absence of inherited antigenic substances on the surface of red blood cells (RBCs). These antigens may be proteins, carbohydrates, glycoproteins, or glycolipids, depending on the blood group system, and some of these antigens are also present on the surface of other types of cells of various tissues. Several of these red blood cell surface antigens, that stem from one allele (or very closely linked genes), collectively form a blood group system.
Prescription drug	A Prescription drug is a licensed medicine that is regulated by legislation to require a prescription before it can be obtained. The term is used to distinguish it from over-the-counter drugs which can be obtained without a prescription. Different jurisdictions have different definitions of what constitutes a Prescription drug.
Fetal alcohol syndrome	Fetal/Foetal alcohol syndrome is a pattern of mental and physical defects that can develop in a fetus when a woman drinks alcohol during pregnancy. The timing and frequency of alcohol consumption during pregnancy are major factors in the risk of a child developing fetal alcohol syndrome. While the ingestion of alcohol does not always result in Fetal alcohol syndrome, there are no medically established guidelines for safe levels of alcohol consumption during pregnancy.
Amniotic fluid	Amniotic fluid or liquor amnii is the nourishing and protecting liquid contained by the amniotic sac of a pregnant woman. The amniotic sac grows and begins to fill, mainly with water, around two weeks after fertilization. After a further 10 weeks the liquid contains proteins, carbohydrates, lipids and phospholipids, urea and electrolytes, all of which aid in the growth of the fetus.
Data collection	Data collection is a term used to describe a process of preparing and collecting data - for example as part of a process improvement or similar project. The purpose of Data collection is to obtain information to keep on record, to make decisions about important issues, to pass information on to others. Primarily, data is collected to provide information regarding a specific topic. Data collection usually takes place early on in an improvement project, and is often formalised through a Data collection plan which often contains the following activity. · Pre collection activity - Agree goals, target data, definitions, methods· Collection - Data collection

Chapter 16. The Prenatal Period,

Smoking cessation	Smoking cessation is the action leading towards the discontinuation of the consumption of a smoked substance, mainly tobacco, but it may encompass cannabis and other substances as well.
	Smoking certain substances can be addictive. This encompasses both psychological and biological addiction.
Home birth	A Home birth is a birth that is planned to occur at home. It is contrasted to birth that occur in a hospital or a birth centre.
	Homebirths are divided into two types -- attended and unattended births.

1. The circulatory system is an organ system that passes nutrients (such as amino acids and electrolytes), gases, hormones, blood cells, etc. to and from cells in the body to help fight diseases and help stabilize body temperature and pH to maintain homeostasis. This system may be seen strictly as a blood distribution network, but some consider the circulatory system as composed of the _____, which distributes blood, and the lymphatic system, which distributes lymph.

   a. Pulmonary circulation
   b. Right ventricle
   c. Systemic circulation
   d. Cardiovascular system

2. The _____'s function is to allow gas exchange to all parts of the body. The space between the alveoli and the capillaries, the anatomy or structure of the exchange system, and the precise physiological uses of the exchanged gases vary depending on the organism. In humans and other mammals, for example, the anatomical features of the _____ include airways, lungs, and the respiratory muscles.

   a. Respiratory system
   b. Forehead
   c. Gingiva
   d. Buccal cavity

3. . _____ refers to how much work is being done when exercising. The intensity has an effect on what fuel the body uses and what kind of adaptations the body makes after exercise (i.e., the training effect).

   Fuel used

   The body uses different amounts of fuels (carbohydrate or fat) depending on the intensity and heart rate.

a. Exercise intensity
b. Exercise prescription software
c. Exertion
d. Explosive exercise

4. _____ refers to the medical and nursing care recommended for women before and during pregnancy. The aim of good _____ is to detect any potential problems early, to prevent them if possible (through recommendations on adequate nutrition, exercise, vitamin intake etc), and to direct the woman to appropriate specialists, hospitals, etc. if necessary.

a. Biotransformation
b. Body water
c. Prenatal care
d. Cerebral edema

5. _____ is a medical procedure used in prenatal diagnosis of chromosomal abnormalities and fetal infections , in which a small amount of amniotic fluid, which contains fetal tissues, is extracted from the amnion or amniotic sac surrounding a developing fetus, and the fetal DNA is examined for genetic abnormalities.

Before the start of the procedure, a local anesthetic can be given to the mother in order to relieve the pain felt during the insertion of the needle used to withdraw the fluid. After the local is in effect, a needle is usually inserted through the mother's abdominal wall, then through the wall of the uterus, and finally into the amniotic sac.

a. abdominal exam
b. Koilonychia
c. Amniocentesis
d. Velopharyngeal inadequacy

1. d
2. a
3. a
4. c
5. c

You can take the complete Chapter Practice Test

for Chapter 16. The Prenatal Period,
on all key terms, persons, places, and concepts.

Online 99 Cents

http://www.epub1625.32.20273.16.cram101.com/

Use www.Cram101.com for all your study needs

including Cram101's online interactive problem solving labs in

chemistry, statistics, mathematics, and more.

Chapter 17. Infant,

Developmental disability

Iron deficiency

Mortality rate

Cognitive development

Denver Developmental Screening Test

Growth chart

Genetic counseling

Down syndrome

Milk allergy

Nutrition

Breast self-examination

Sudden infant death syndrome

Child abuse

Prevention

Male circumcision

Prescription drug

Genetic variation

Lead poisoning

Health effect

CHAPTER OUTLINE: KEY TERMS, PEOPLE, PLACES, CONCEPTS

	Heat stroke
	Motor skills
	Day care
	Data collection
	Risk factor
	Health care

CHAPTER HIGHLIGHTS & NOTES: KEY TERMS, PEOPLE, PLACES, CONCEPTS

| Developmental disability | Developmental disability is a term used in the United States and Canada to describe life-long disabilities attributable to mental and/or physical impairments, manifested prior to age 18. It is not synonymous with 'developmental delay' which is often a consequence of a temporary illness or trauma during childhood.

Terminology and history

The term is used most commonly in the U.S. and Canada to refer to disabilities affecting daily functioning in three or more of the following areas: capacity for independent living, economic self-sufficiency, learning, mobility, receptive and expressive language, self-care, and self-direction.

The term first appeared in U.S. law in 1970, when Congress used the term to describe the population of individuals who had historically been placed in state institutions, in its effort to improve conditions in these dehumanizing facilities (P.L. 91-517, 'The Developmental Disabilities Services and Facilities Construction Act of 1970'). |
| --- | --- |
| Iron deficiency | Iron deficiency is one of the most commonly known forms of nutritional deficiencies. |

Chapter 17. Infant,

	In the human body, iron is present in all cells and has several vital functions--as a carrier of oxygen to the tissues from the lungs in the form of hemoglobin, as a transport medium for electrons within the cells in the form of cytochromes, and as an integral part of enzyme reactions in various tissues. Too little iron can interfere with these vital functions and lead to morbidity and mortality.
Mortality rate	Mortality rate is a measure of the number of deaths (in general,) in some population, scaled to the size of that population, per unit time. Mortality rate is typically expressed in units of deaths per 1000 individuals per year; thus, a Mortality rate of 9.5 in a population of 100,000 would mean 950 deaths per year in that entire population. It is distinct from morbidity rate, which refers to the number of individuals in poor health during a given time period (the prevalence rate) or the number who currently have that disease (the incidence rate), scaled to the size of the population.
Cognitive development	Cognitive development is a field of study in neuroscience and psychology focusing on a child's development in terms of information processing, conceptual resources, perceptual skill, language learning, and other aspects of brain development and cognitive psychology. A large portion of research has gone into understanding how a child conceptualizes the world. Jean Piaget was a major force in the founding of this field, forming his 'theory of Cognitive development'.
Denver Developmental Screening Test	The Denver Developmental Screening Test , commonly known as the Denver Scale, is a test for screening cognitive and behavioural problems in preschool children. It was developed by William K. Frankenburg and first introduced by him and J.B. Dobbs in 1967. The test is currently marketed by Denver Developmental Materials, Inc., in Denver, Colorado, hence the name.
Growth chart	A Growth chart is used by pediatricians and other health care providers to follow a child's growth over time. Growth charts have been constructed by observing the growth of large numbers of normal children over time. The height, weight, and head circumference of a child can be compared to the expected parameters of children of the same age and sex to determine whether the child is growing appropriately.
Genetic counseling	Genetic counseling is the process by which patients or relatives, at risk of an inherited disorder, are advised of the consequences and nature of the disorder, the probability of developing or transmitting it, and the options open to them in management and family planning in order to prevent, avoid or ameliorate it. This complex process can be seen from diagnostic (the actual estimation of risk) and supportive aspects.

A genetic counselor is a medical genetics expert with a master of science degree. |
| Down syndrome | Down syndrome, trisomy 21, is a chromosomal condition caused by the presence of all or part of an extra 21st chromosome. |

It is named after John Langdon Down, the British physician who described the syndrome in 1866. The condition was identified as a chromosome 21 trisomy by Jérôme Lejeune in 1959. Down syndrome in a fetus can be identified with amniocentesis (with risks of fetal injury and/or miscarriage) during pregnancy, or in a baby at birth.

Down syndrome is a chromosomal condition characterized by the presence of an extra copy of genetic material on the 21st chromosome, either in whole (trisomy 21) or part (such as due to translocations).

| Milk allergy | Milk allergy is a food allergy immune adverse reaction to one or more of the proteins in cow's milk.

The principal symptoms are gastrointestinal, dermatological and respiratory. These can translate to: skin rash, hives, vomiting, diarrhea, constipation and distress. |

Nutrition — Nutrition is the provision, to cells and organisms, of the materials necessary (in the form of food) to support life. Many common health problems can be prevented or alleviated with a healthy diet.

The diet of an organism is what it eats, and is largely determined by the perceived palatability of foods.

Breast self-examination — Breast self-examination (Breast self-examinationE) is a method of finding abnormalities of the breast, for early detection of breast cancer. The method involves the woman herself looking at and feeling each breast for possible lumps, distortions or swelling.

Breast self-examinationE was once promoted heavily as a means of finding cancer at a more curable stage, but randomized controlled studies found that it was not effective in preventing death, and actually caused harm through needless biopsies and surgery.

Sudden infant death syndrome — Sudden infant death syndrome is a syndrome marked by the sudden death of an infant that is unexpected by history and remains unexplained after a thorough forensic autopsy and a detailed death scene investigation. It is still sometimes referred to by the former terms cot death (in the United Kingdom, Ireland, Australia, India, South Africa and New Zealand) or crib death (in North America).

Typically the infant is found dead after having been put to bed, and exhibits no signs of having suffered.

Child abuse — Child abuse is the physical or psychological/emotional mistreatment of children.

Chapter 17. Infant,

In the United States, the Centers for Disease Control and Prevention (CDC) define child maltreatment as any act or series of acts of commission or omission by a parent or other caregiver that results in harm, potential for harm, or threat of harm to a child. Most Child abuse occurs in a child's home, with a smaller amount occurring in the organizations, schools or communities the child interacts with.

| Prevention | Prevention refers to:

· Preventive medicine · Hazard Prevention, the process of risk study and elimination and mitigation in emergency management · Risk Prevention · Risk management · Preventive maintenance · Crime Prevention

· Prevention, an album by Scottish band De Rosa · Prevention a magazine about health in the United States · Prevent (company), a textile company from Slovenia

| Male circumcision | It has been variously proposed that male circumcision began as a religious sacrifice, as a rite of passage marking a boy's entrance into adulthood, as a form of sympathetic magic to ensure virility, as a means of suppressing or enhancing sexual pleasure, as an aid to hygiene where regular bathing was impractical, as a means of marking those of lower or higher social status, as a means of differentiating a circumcising group from their non-circumcising neighbors, as a means of discouraging masturbation or other socially proscribed sexual behaviors, to remove 'excess' pleasure, to increase a man's attractiveness to women, as a symbolic castration, as a demonstration of one's ability to endure pain, or as a male counterpart to menstruation or the breaking of the hymen or to copy the rare natural occurrence of a missing foreskin of an important leader. It has been suggested that the custom of circumcision gave advantages to tribes that practiced it and thus led to its spread regardless of whether the people understood this. It is possible that circumcision arose independently in different cultures for different reasons.

| Prescription drug | A Prescription drug is a licensed medicine that is regulated by legislation to require a prescription before it can be obtained. The term is used to distinguish it from over-the-counter drugs which can be obtained without a prescription. Different jurisdictions have different definitions of what constitutes a Prescription drug.

| Genetic variation | Genetic variation, variation in alleles of genes, occurs both within and among populations. Genetic variation is important because it provides the 'raw material' for natural selection.

Genetic variation among individuals within a population can be identified at a variety of levels.

| Lead poisoning | Lead poisoning is a medical condition caused by increased levels of the heavy metal lead in the body.

Lead interferes with a variety of body processes and is toxic to many organs and tissues including the heart, bones, intestines, kidneys, and reproductive and nervous systems. It interferes with the development of the nervous system and is therefore particularly toxic to children, causing potentially permanent learning and behavior disorders.

Health effect

Health effects are changes in health resulting from exposure to a source. Health effects are an important consideration in many areas, such as hygiene, pollution studies, workplace safety, nutrition and health sciences in general. Some of the major environmental sources of Health effects are air pollution, water pollution, soil contamination, noise pollution and over-illumination.

Heat stroke

Heat stroke is defined as a temperature of greater than 40.6 °C (105.1 °F) due to environmental heat exposure with lack of thermoregulation. This is distinct from a fever, where there is a physiological increase in the temperature set point of the body.

Treatment involves rapid mechanical cooling.

A number of heat illnesses exist including:

· Heat stroke as defined by a temperature of greater than >40.6 °C (105.1 °F) due to environmental heat exposure with lack of thermoregulation. · Heat exhaustion · Heat syncope · Heat edema · Heat cramps · Heat tetany

Heat stroke presents with a hyperthermia of greater than >40.6 °C (105.1 °F) in combination with confusion and a lack of sweating.

Motor skills

A motor skill is a learned sequence of movements that combine to produce a smooth, efficient action in order to master a particular task.

· Gross Motor skills include lifting one's head, rolling over, sitting up, balancing, crawling, and walking. Gross motor development usually follows a pattern. Generally large muscles develop before smaller ones, thus, gross motor development is the foundation for developing skills in other areas (such as fine Motor skills).

Day care

Day care or child care is care of a child during the day by a person other than the child's legal guardians, typically performed by someone outside the child's immediate family. Day care is typically an ongoing service during specific periods, such as the parents' time at work.

The service is known as child care in the United Kingdom and Australia and Day care in North America (although childcare also has a broader meaning).

Chapter 17. Infant,

Data collection	Data collection is a term used to describe a process of preparing and collecting data - for example as part of a process improvement or similar project. The purpose of Data collection is to obtain information to keep on record, to make decisions about important issues, to pass information on to others. Primarily, data is collected to provide information regarding a specific topic.
	Data collection usually takes place early on in an improvement project, and is often formalised through a Data collection plan which often contains the following activity.
	· Pre collection activity - Agree goals, target data, definitions, methods· Collection - Data collection· Present Findings - usually involves some form of sorting analysis and/or presentation.
Risk factor	A Risk factor is a variable associated with an increased risk of disease or infection. Risk factors are correlational and not necessarily causal, because correlation does not imply causation. For example, being young cannot be said to cause measles, but young people are more at risk as they are less likely to have developed immunity during a previous epidemic.
Health care	Health care , refers to the treatment and management of illness, and the preservation of health through services offered by the medical, dental, complementary and alternative medicine, pharmaceutical, clinical laboratory sciences , nursing, and allied health professions. Health care embraces all the goods and services designed to promote health, including 'preventive, curative and palliative interventions, whether directed to individuals or to populations'.
	Before the term Health care became popular, English-speakers referred to medicine or to the health sector and spoke of the treatment and prevention of illness and disease.

Chapter 17. Infant,

1. _____ is a term used in the United States and Canada to describe life-long disabilities attributable to mental and/or physical impairments, manifested prior to age 18. It is not synonymous with 'developmental delay' which is often a consequence of a temporary illness or trauma during childhood.

Terminology and history

The term is used most commonly in the U.S. and Canada to refer to disabilities affecting daily functioning in three or more of the following areas: capacity for independent living, economic self-sufficiency, learning, mobility, receptive and expressive language, self-care, and self-direction.

The term first appeared in U.S. law in 1970, when Congress used the term to describe the population of individuals who had historically been placed in state institutions, in its effort to improve conditions in these dehumanizing facilities (P.L. 91-517, 'The Developmental Disabilities Services and Facilities Construction Act of 1970').

a. Developmental disability
b. The Council on Quality and Leadership
c. Developmental dysfluency
d. Direct support professional

2. _____ is defined as a temperature of greater than 40.6 °C (105.1 °F) due to environmental heat exposure with lack of thermoregulation. This is distinct from a fever, where there is a physiological increase in the temperature set point of the body.

Treatment involves rapid mechanical cooling.

A number of heat illnesses exist including:

· _____ as defined by a temperature of greater than >40.6 °C (105.1 °F) due to environmental heat exposure with lack of thermoregulation. · Heat exhaustion · Heat syncope · Heat edema · Heat cramps · Heat tetany

_____ presents with a hyperthermia of greater than >40.6 °C (105.1 °F) in combination with confusion and a lack of sweating.

a. Bacteriophage
b. Blue Zone
c. Communities That Care
d. Heat stroke

3. . _____ is a field of study in neuroscience and psychology focusing on a child's development in terms of information processing, conceptual resources, perceptual skill, language learning, and other aspects of brain development and cognitive psychology. A large portion of research has gone into understanding how a child conceptualizes the world. Jean Piaget was a major force in the founding of this field, forming his 'theory of _____'.

a. Bacteriophage
b. Cognitive development

Chapter 17. Infant,

c. Developmental dysfluency

d. Direct support professional

4. A motor skill is a learned sequence of movements that combine to produce a smooth, efficient action in order to master a particular task.

· Gross _____ include lifting one's head, rolling over, sitting up, balancing, crawling, and walking. Gross motor development usually follows a pattern. Generally large muscles develop before smaller ones, thus, gross motor development is the foundation for developing skills in other areas (such as fine _____).

a. abdominal exam

b. Motor skills

c. Communities That Care

d. Deconditioning

5. _____s are changes in health resulting from exposure to a source. _____s are an important consideration in many areas, such as hygiene, pollution studies, workplace safety, nutrition and health sciences in general. Some of the major environmental sources of _____s are air pollution, water pollution, soil contamination, noise pollution and over-illumination.

a. Health effector

b. Blue Zone

c. Health effect

d. Deconditioning

1. a
2. d
3. b
4. b
5. c

You can take the complete Chapter Practice Test

for Chapter 17. Infant,
on all key terms, persons, places, and concepts.

Online 99 Cents

http://www.epub1625.32.20273.17.cram101.com/

Use www.Cram101.com for all your study needs

including Cram101's online interactive problem solving labs in

chemistry, statistics, mathematics, and more.

Chapter 18. Toddler,

Toddler

Respiratory tract

Endocrine system

Toilet training

Cognitive development

Language development

Otitis media

Child abuse

Risk factor

Vitamin D

Motor skills

Day care

Lead poisoning

Case study

Health care

Staphylococcus aureus

Chapter 18. Toddler,

Toddler	A Toddler is a young child who is of the age of learning to walk, between infancy and childhood. Toddling usually begins between age 12 and 24 months. During the Toddler stage, the child also learns a great deal about social roles, develops motor skills, and first starts to use language.
Respiratory tract	In humans the Respiratory tract is the part of the anatomy that has to do with the process of respiration.
	The Respiratory tract is divided into 3 segments:
	· Upper Respiratory tract: nose and nasal passages, paranasal sinuses, and throat or pharynx · Respiratory airways: voice box or larynx, trachea, bronchi, and bronchioles · Lungs: respiratory bronchioles, alveolar ducts, alveolar sacs, and alveoli
	The Respiratory tract is a common site for infections. Upper Respiratory tract infections are probably the most common infections in the world.
	Most of the Respiratory tract exists merely as a piping system for air to travel in the lungs; alveoli are the only part of the lung that exchanges oxygen and carbon dioxide with the blood.
Endocrine system	The Endocrine system is a system of glands, each of which secretes a type of hormone to regulate the body. The field of study that deals with disorders of endocrine glands is endocrinology, a branch of the wider field of internal medicine. The Endocrine system is an information signal system much like the nervous system.
Toilet training	Toilet training, or potty training, is the process of training a young child to use the toilet for urination and defecation, though training may start with a smaller toilet bowl-shaped device (often known as a potty). In Western countries it is usually started and completed between the ages of 12 months and three years with boys typically being at the higher end of the age spectrum.
	Cultural factors play a large part in what age is deemed appropriate, with the age being generally later in America.
	Most advise that Toilet training is a mutual task, requiring cooperation, agreement and understanding between child and the caregiver, and the best potty training techniques emphasize consistency and positive reinforcement over punishment - making it fun for the child.
Cognitive development	Cognitive development is a field of study in neuroscience and psychology focusing on a child's development in terms of information processing, conceptual resources, perceptual skill, language learning, and other aspects of brain development and cognitive psychology.

A large portion of research has gone into understanding how a child conceptualizes the world. Jean Piaget was a major force in the founding of this field, forming his 'theory of Cognitive development'.

Language development	Language development is a process starting early in human life, when a person begins to acquire language by learning it as it is spoken and by mimicry. Children's language development moves from simple to complex. Infants start without language.
Otitis media	Otitis media is inflammation of the middle ear, or middle ear infection. Otitis media occurs in the area between the ear drum and the inner ear, including a duct known as the eustachian tube. It is one of the two categories of ear inflammation that can underlie what is commonly called an earache, the other being otitis externa.
Child abuse	Child abuse is the physical or psychological/emotional mistreatment of children. In the United States, the Centers for Disease Control and Prevention (CDC) define child maltreatment as any act or series of acts of commission or omission by a parent or other caregiver that results in harm, potential for harm, or threat of harm to a child. Most Child abuse occurs in a child's home, with a smaller amount occurring in the organizations, schools or communities the child interacts with.
Risk factor	A Risk factor is a variable associated with an increased risk of disease or infection. Risk factors are correlational and not necessarily causal, because correlation does not imply causation. For example, being young cannot be said to cause measles, but young people are more at risk as they are less likely to have developed immunity during a previous epidemic.
Vitamin D	Vitamin D is a group of fat-soluble prohormones, the two major forms of which are Vitamin D_2 (or ergocalciferol) and Vitamin D_3 (or cholecalciferol). Vitamin D obtained from sun exposure, food, and supplements, is biologically inert and must undergo two hydroxylation reactions to be activated in the body. Calcitriol (1,25-Dihydroxycholecalciferol) is the active form of Vitamin D found in the body.
Motor skills	A motor skill is a learned sequence of movements that combine to produce a smooth, efficient action in order to master a particular task. · Gross Motor skills include lifting one's head, rolling over, sitting up, balancing, crawling, and walking. Gross motor development usually follows a pattern. Generally large muscles develop before smaller ones, thus, gross motor development is the foundation for developing skills in other areas (such as fine Motor skills).

Day care	Day care or child care is care of a child during the day by a person other than the child's legal guardians, typically performed by someone outside the child's immediate family. Day care is typically an ongoing service during specific periods, such as the parents' time at work.
	The service is known as child care in the United Kingdom and Australia and Day care in North America (although childcare also has a broader meaning).
Lead poisoning	Lead poisoning is a medical condition caused by increased levels of the heavy metal lead in the body. Lead interferes with a variety of body processes and is toxic to many organs and tissues including the heart, bones, intestines, kidneys, and reproductive and nervous systems. It interferes with the development of the nervous system and is therefore particularly toxic to children, causing potentially permanent learning and behavior disorders.
Case study	A Case study is a research methodology common in social science. It is based on an in-depth investigation of a single individual, group, or event to explore causation in order to find underlying principles.
Health care	Health care , refers to the treatment and management of illness, and the preservation of health through services offered by the medical, dental, complementary and alternative medicine, pharmaceutical, clinical laboratory sciences , nursing, and allied health professions. Health care embraces all the goods and services designed to promote health, including 'preventive, curative and palliative interventions, whether directed to individuals or to populations'.
	Before the term Health care became popular, English-speakers referred to medicine or to the health sector and spoke of the treatment and prevention of illness and disease.
Staphylococcus aureus	Staphylococcus aureus is a facultatively anaerobic, gram positive coccus and is the most common cause of staph infections. It is a spherical bacterium, frequently part of the skin flora found in the nose and on skin. About 20% of the population are long-term carriers of S. aureus.

Chapter 18. Toddler,

1. _____ is a process starting early in human life, when a person begins to acquire language by learning it as it is spoken and by mimicry. Children's _____ moves from simple to complex. Infants start without language.

    a. Stuttering
    b. Logographic cues
    c. Phonological awareness
    d. Language development

2. A motor skill is a learned sequence of movements that combine to produce a smooth, efficient action in order to master a particular task.

    · Gross _____ include lifting one's head, rolling over, sitting up, balancing, crawling, and walking. Gross motor development usually follows a pattern. Generally large muscles develop before smaller ones, thus, gross motor development is the foundation for developing skills in other areas (such as fine _____).

    a. abdominal exam
    b. Achilles tendon
    c. Motor skills
    d. Adenoviridae

3. A _____ is a young child who is of the age of learning to walk, between infancy and childhood. Toddling usually begins between age 12 and 24 months. During the _____ stage, the child also learns a great deal about social roles, develops motor skills, and first starts to use language.

    a. Toddler
    b. Baroreflex
    c. Benign prostatic hyperplasia
    d. Benzathine benzylpenicillin

4. _____ is a medical condition caused by increased levels of the heavy metal lead in the body. Lead interferes with a variety of body processes and is toxic to many organs and tissues including the heart, bones, intestines, kidneys, and reproductive and nervous systems. It interferes with the development of the nervous system and is therefore particularly toxic to children, causing potentially permanent learning and behavior disorders.

    a. Lead poisoning
    b. Baroreflex
    c. Benign prostatic hyperplasia
    d. Benzathine benzylpenicillin

5. . _____ is the physical or psychological/emotional mistreatment of children. In the United States, the Centers for Disease Control and Prevention (CDC) define child maltreatment as any act or series of acts of commission or omission by a parent or other caregiver that results in harm, potential for harm, or threat of harm to a child. Most _____ occurs in a child's home, with a smaller amount occurring in the organizations, schools or communities the child interacts with.

    a. Bacteriophage

Chapter 18. Toddler,

Visit Cram101.com for full Practice Exams

b. Child abuse

c. Phonological awareness

d. Representational systems

1. d
2. c
3. a
4. a
5. b

You can take the complete Chapter Practice Test

for Chapter 18. Toddler,
on all key terms, persons, places, and concepts.

Online 99 Cents

http://www.epub1625.32.20273.18.cram101.com/

Use www.Cram101.com for all your study needs

including Cram101's online interactive problem solving labs in

chemistry, statistics, mathematics, and more.

	Growth failure
	Sweat glands
	Cardiovascular system
	Immune system
	Otitis media
	Cystic fibrosis
	Muscular dystrophy
	Musculoskeletal system
	Nervous system
	Developmental milestones
	Dental caries
	Food allergy
	Milk allergy
	Cognitive development
	Color blindness
	Strabismus
	Smoking
	Language development
	Human development

Chapter 19. Preschool Child,

_____ | Child abuse

_____ | Risk factor

_____ | Lead poisoning

_____ | Cancer

_____ | Case study

_____ | Data collection

_____ | Health care

_____ | Health promotion

CHAPTER HIGHLIGHTS & NOTES: KEY TERMS, PEOPLE, PLACES, CONCEPTS

Growth failure	Growth failure is a medical term for a rate of a child's growth which is poorer than normal for age, sex, stage of maturation, and genetic height expectation. Growth failure usually has an abnormal cause or causes. Many short children are growing normally and this is not referred to as growth failure.
Sweat glands	Sweat glands also refered to as sudoriferous glands are exocrine glands, found under the skin of all mammal species, that are used for body temperature regulation. In humans a system of apocrine - and merocrine Sweat glands is the main method of cooling. Many other mammals rely on panting or other means as a primary source of cooling, but still use Sweat glands to aid in body temperature regulation.
Cardiovascular system	The circulatory system is an organ system that passes nutrients (such as amino acids and electrolytes), gases, hormones, blood cells, etc. to and from cells in the body to help fight diseases and help stabilize body temperature and pH to maintain homeostasis.

Immune system	An immune system is a system of biological structures and processes within an organism that protects against disease by identifying and killing pathogens and tumour cells. It detects a wide variety of agents, from viruses to parasitic worms, and needs to distinguish them from the organism's own healthy cells and tissues in order to function properly. Detection is complicated as pathogens can evolve rapidly, producing adaptations that avoid the immune system and allow the pathogens to successfully infect their hosts.
Otitis media	Otitis media is inflammation of the middle ear, or middle ear infection. Otitis media occurs in the area between the ear drum and the inner ear, including a duct known as the eustachian tube. It is one of the two categories of ear inflammation that can underlie what is commonly called an earache, the other being otitis externa.
Cystic fibrosis	Cystic fibrosis is a common recessive genetic disease which affects the entire body, causing progressive disability and often early death. The name cystic fibrosis refers to the characteristic scarring (fibrosis) and cyst formation within the pancreas, first recognized in the 1930s. Difficulty breathing is the most serious symptom and results from frequent lung infections that are treated with, though not cured by, antibiotics and other medications.
Muscular dystrophy	Muscular dystrophy refers to a group of hereditary muscle diseases that weaken the muscles that move the human body. Muscular dystrophies are characterized by progressive skeletal muscle weakness, defects in muscle proteins, and the death of muscle cells and tissue. Nine diseases including Duchenne, Becker, limb girdle, congenital, facioscapulohumeral, myotonic, oculopharyngeal, distal, and Emery-Dreifuss are always classified as muscular dystrophy but there are more than 100 diseases in total with similarities to muscular dystrophy.
Musculoskeletal system	A Musculoskeletal system is an organ system that gives animals (including humans) the ability to move using the muscular and skeletal systems. The Musculoskeletal system provides form, stability, and movement to the body. It is made up of the body's bones (the skeleton), muscles, cartilage, tendons, ligaments, joints, and other connective tissue (the tissue that supports and binds tissues and organs together).
Nervous system	The Nervous system is an organ system containing a network of specialized cells called neurons that coordinate the actions of an animal and transmit signals between different parts of its body. In most animals the Nervous system consists of two parts, central and peripheral. The central Nervous system contains the brain and spinal cord.
Developmental milestones	Developmental milestones are tasks most children learn that commonly appear in certain age ranges. For example:

· Ability to lift and control the orientation of the head (Neck control) is attained at about 3 months · Crawling begins at about 7 months · Walking unsupported is attained at about 12 months · Speech begins · Voice lowers in pitch (especially noticeable in boys) · Pubic hair appears · Genitals and reproductive organs mature · Menses begin (females) · Body hair and facial hair appears

'Normal' age ranges for many milestones are broad . For this and other reasons, a single delayed milestone, especially task-related, is rarely in itself a basis for diagnosing a problem.

Dental caries	Dental caries is a disease wherein bacterial processes damage hard tooth structure. These tissues progressively break down, producing dental cavities. Two groups of bacteria are responsible for initiating caries: Streptococcus mutans and Lactobacilli.
Food allergy	A Food allergy is an adverse immune response to a food protein. Food allergy is distinct from other adverse responses to food, such as food intolerance, pharmacologic reactions, and toxin-mediated reactions. The food protein triggering the allergic response is termed a food allergen.
Milk allergy	Milk allergy is a food allergy immune adverse reaction to one or more of the proteins in cow's milk. The principal symptoms are gastrointestinal, dermatological and respiratory. These can translate to: skin rash, hives, vomiting, diarrhea, constipation and distress.
Cognitive development	Cognitive development is a field of study in neuroscience and psychology focusing on a child's development in terms of information processing, conceptual resources, perceptual skill, language learning, and other aspects of brain development and cognitive psychology. A large portion of research has gone into understanding how a child conceptualizes the world. Jean Piaget was a major force in the founding of this field, forming his 'theory of Cognitive development'.
Color blindness	Color blindness is the decreased ability to perceive differences between some of the colors that others can distinguish. It is most often of genetic nature, but may also occur because of some eye, nerve, or brain damage, or exposure to certain chemicals. The English chemist John Dalton published the first scientific paper on this subject in 1798, 'Extraordinary facts relating to the vision of colours', after the realization of his own color blindness.
Strabismus	Strabismus is a condition in which the eyes are not properly aligned with each other.

	It typically involves a lack of coordination between the extraocular muscles that prevents bringing the gaze of each eye to the same point in space and preventing proper binocular vision, which may adversely affect depth perception. Strabismus can be either a disorder of the brain in coordinating the eyes, or of one or more of the relevant muscles' power or direction of motion.
Smoking	Smoking is a practice in which a substance, most commonly tobacco, is burned and the smoke tasted or inhaled. This is primarily practised as a route of administration for recreational drug use, as combustion releases the active substances in drugs such as nicotine and makes them available for absorption through the lungs. It can also be done as a part of rituals, to induce trances and spiritual enlightenment.
Language development	Language development is a process starting early in human life, when a person begins to acquire language by learning it as it is spoken and by mimicry. Children's language development moves from simple to complex. Infants start without language.
Human development	Human development is the process of growing to maturity. In biological terms, this entails growth from a one-celled zygote to an adult human being. Development begins with fertilization, the process by which the male gamete, the sperm cell, and the female gamete, the egg, fuse to produce a zygote.
Child abuse	Child abuse is the physical or psychological/emotional mistreatment of children. In the United States, the Centers for Disease Control and Prevention (CDC) define child maltreatment as any act or series of acts of commission or omission by a parent or other caregiver that results in harm, potential for harm, or threat of harm to a child. Most Child abuse occurs in a child's home, with a smaller amount occurring in the organizations, schools or communities the child interacts with.
Risk factor	A Risk factor is a variable associated with an increased risk of disease or infection. Risk factors are correlational and not necessarily causal, because correlation does not imply causation. For example, being young cannot be said to cause measles, but young people are more at risk as they are less likely to have developed immunity during a previous epidemic.
Lead poisoning	Lead poisoning is a medical condition caused by increased levels of the heavy metal lead in the body. Lead interferes with a variety of body processes and is toxic to many organs and tissues including the heart, bones, intestines, kidneys, and reproductive and nervous systems. It interferes with the development of the nervous system and is therefore particularly toxic to children, causing potentially permanent learning and behavior disorders.
Cancer	Cancer

(medical term: malignant neoplasm) is a class of diseases in which a group of cells display uncontrolled growth, invasion that intrudes upon and destroys adjacent tissues, and sometimes metastasis, or spreading to other locations in the body via lymph or blood. These three malignant properties of cancers differentiate them from benign tumors, which do not invade or metastasize.

Researchers divide the causes of cancer into two groups: those with an environmental cause and those with a hereditary genetic cause.

Case study	A Case study is a research methodology common in social science. It is based on an in-depth investigation of a single individual, group, or event to explore causation in order to find underlying principles.
Data collection	Data collection is a term used to describe a process of preparing and collecting data - for example as part of a process improvement or similar project. The purpose of Data collection is to obtain information to keep on record, to make decisions about important issues, to pass information on to others. Primarily, data is collected to provide information regarding a specific topic. Data collection usually takes place early on in an improvement project, and is often formalised through a Data collection plan which often contains the following activity. · Pre collection activity - Agree goals, target data, definitions, methods· Collection - Data collection· Present Findings - usually involves some form of sorting analysis and/or presentation.
Health care	Health care , refers to the treatment and management of illness, and the preservation of health through services offered by the medical, dental, complementary and alternative medicine, pharmaceutical, clinical laboratory sciences , nursing, and allied health professions. Health care embraces all the goods and services designed to promote health, including 'preventive, curative and palliative interventions, whether directed to individuals or to populations'. Before the term Health care became popular, English-speakers referred to medicine or to the health sector and spoke of the treatment and prevention of illness and disease.
Health promotion	Health promotion has been defined by the World Health Organization's 2005 Bangkok Charter for Health promotion in a Globalized World as 'the process of enabling people to increase control over their health and its determinants, and thereby improve their health'. The primary means of Health promotion occur through developing healthy public policy that addresses the prerequisities of health such as income, housing, food security, employment, and quality working conditions.

1. A _____ is an organ system that gives animals (including humans) the ability to move using the muscular and skeletal systems. The _____ provides form, stability, and movement to the body.

It is made up of the body's bones (the skeleton), muscles, cartilage, tendons, ligaments, joints, and other connective tissue (the tissue that supports and binds tissues and organs together).

a. Plantarflexion
b. Musculoskeletal system
c. Flexion
d. Bacteriophage

2. _____ is a process starting early in human life, when a person begins to acquire language by learning it as it is spoken and by mimicry. Children's _____ moves from simple to complex. Infants start without language.

a. Language development
b. Logographic cues
c. Phonological awareness
d. Representational systems

3. _____ is a medical term for a rate of a child's growth which is poorer than normal for age, sex, stage of maturation, and genetic height expectation. _____ usually has an abnormal cause or causes. Many short children are growing normally and this is not referred to as _____.

a. Breastfeeding
b. Mark Lester
c. Growth failure
d. Preterm birth

4. The circulatory system is an organ system that passes nutrients (such as amino acids and electrolytes), gases, hormones, blood cells, etc. to and from cells in the body to help fight diseases and help stabilize body temperature and pH to maintain homeostasis. This system may be seen strictly as a blood distribution network, but some consider the circulatory system as composed of the _____, which distributes blood, and the lymphatic system, which distributes lymph.

a. Pulmonary circulation
b. Cardiovascular system
c. Systemic circulation
d. Vein

5. . An _____ is a system of biological structures and processes within an organism that protects against disease by identifying and killing pathogens and tumour cells. It detects a wide variety of agents, from viruses to parasitic worms, and needs to distinguish them from the organism's own healthy cells and tissues in order to function properly. Detection is complicated as pathogens can evolve rapidly, producing adaptations that avoid the _____ and allow the pathogens to successfully infect their hosts.

a. Immune system

b. adaptive immune system

c. Antigen

d. Immunoglobulin A

ANSWER KEY
Chapter 19. Preschool Child,

1. b
2. a
3. c
4. b
5. a

You can take the complete Chapter Practice Test

for Chapter 19. Preschool Child,
on all key terms, persons, places, and concepts.

Online 99 Cents

http://www.epub1625.32.20273.19.cram101.com/

Use www.Cram101.com for all your study needs

including Cram101's online interactive problem solving labs in

chemistry, statistics, mathematics, and more.

CHAPTER OUTLINE: KEY TERMS, PEOPLE, PLACES, CONCEPTS

	Heart rate
	Immune system
	Exercise intensity
	Growth chart
	Blood pressure
	Deciduous teeth
	Dental caries
	Musculoskeletal system
	Periodontal disease
	Sleep apnea
	Cognitive development
	Hyperopia
	Otitis media
	Smoking
	Health promotion
	Kinesthetic learning
	Auditory
	Auditory learning
	Language development

_____ Case study

_____ Learning disability

_____ Individuals with Disabilities Education Act

_____ Human development

_____ Cardiovascular disease

_____ Child abuse

_____ Risk factor

_____ Sex education

_____ Sexual function

_____ Child depression

_____ Symptom

_____ Alcohol abuse

_____ Seat belt

_____ Hepatitis B

_____ Prescription drug

_____ Immunization

_____ Vaccination

_____ Vaccine

_____ Cancer

	Data collection
	Health care
	Health education

Heart rate	Heart rate is the number of heartbeats per unit of time - typically expressed as beats per minute (BPM) - which can vary as the body's need for oxygen changes, such as during exercise or sleep. The measurement of Heart rate is used by medical professionals to assist in the diagnosis and tracking of medical conditions. It is also used by individuals, such as athletes, who are interested in monitoring their Heart rate to gain maximum efficiency from their training.
Immune system	An immune system is a system of biological structures and processes within an organism that protects against disease by identifying and killing pathogens and tumour cells. It detects a wide variety of agents, from viruses to parasitic worms, and needs to distinguish them from the organism's own healthy cells and tissues in order to function properly. Detection is complicated as pathogens can evolve rapidly, producing adaptations that avoid the immune system and allow the pathogens to successfully infect their hosts.
Exercise intensity	Exercise intensity refers to how much work is being done when exercising. The intensity has an effect on what fuel the body uses and what kind of adaptations the body makes after exercise (i.e., the training effect). Fuel used The body uses different amounts of fuels (carbohydrate or fat) depending on the intensity and heart rate.
Growth chart	A Growth chart is used by pediatricians and other health care providers to follow a child's growth over time. Growth charts have been constructed by observing the growth of large numbers of normal children over time.

Chapter 20. School-Age Child,

Blood pressure	Blood pressure is the pressure (force per unit area) exerted by circulating blood on the walls of blood vessels, and constitutes one of the principal vital signs. The pressure of the circulating blood decreases as it moves away from the heart through arteries and capillaries, and toward the heart through veins. When unqualified, the term Blood pressure usually refers to brachial arterial pressure: that is, in the major blood vessel of the upper left or right arm that takes blood away from the heart.
Deciduous teeth	Deciduous teeth, otherwise known as milk teeth, baby teeth, temporary teeth and primary teeth, are the first set of teeth in the growth development of humans and many other mammals. They develop during the embryonic stage of development and erupt--that is, they become visible in the mouth--during infancy. They are usually lost and replaced by permanent teeth, but in the absence of permanent replacements, they can remain functional for many years.
Dental caries	Dental caries is a disease wherein bacterial processes damage hard tooth structure. These tissues progressively break down, producing dental cavities. Two groups of bacteria are responsible for initiating caries: Streptococcus mutans and Lactobacilli.
Musculoskeletal system	A Musculoskeletal system is an organ system that gives animals (including humans) the ability to move using the muscular and skeletal systems. The Musculoskeletal system provides form, stability, and movement to the body. It is made up of the body's bones (the skeleton), muscles, cartilage, tendons, ligaments, joints, and other connective tissue (the tissue that supports and binds tissues and organs together).
Periodontal disease	Periodontal diseases are those diseases that affect one or more of the periodontal tissues: · alveolar bone · periodontal ligament · cementum · gingiva While many different diseases affect the tooth-supporting structures, plaque-induced inflammatory lesions make up the vast majority of Periodontal diseases and have traditionally been divided into two categories: · gingivitis or · periodontitis. While in some sites or individuals, gingivitis never progresses to periodontitis, data indicates that gingivitis always precedes periodontitis. Investigation into the causes and characteristics of Periodontal diseases began in the 18th century with pure clinical observation, and this remained the primary form of investigation well into the 19th century. During this time, the signs and symptoms of Periodontal diseases were firmly established:

	· Rather than a single disease entity, Periodontal disease is a combination of multiple disease processes that share a common clinical manifestation. · The etiology (cause) includes both local and systemic factors. · The disease consists of a chronic inflammation associated with loss of alveolar bone. · Advanced disease features include pus and exudates. · Essential aspects of successful treatment of Periodontal disease include initial debridement and maintenance of proper oral hygiene.
Sleep apnea	Sleep apnea is a sleep disorder characterized by pauses in breathing during sleep. Each episode, called an apnea , from α- (a-), privative, πνîειν (pnéein), to breathe), lasts long enough so that one or more breaths are missed, and such episodes occur repeatedly throughout sleep. The standard definition of any apneic event includes a minimum 10 second interval between breaths, with either a neurological arousal (a 3-second or greater shift in EEG frequency, measured at C3, C4, O1, or O2), a blood oxygen desaturation of 3-4% or greater, or both arousal and desaturation.
Cognitive development	Cognitive development is a field of study in neuroscience and psychology focusing on a child's development in terms of information processing, conceptual resources, perceptual skill, language learning, and other aspects of brain development and cognitive psychology. A large portion of research has gone into understanding how a child conceptualizes the world. Jean Piaget was a major force in the founding of this field, forming his 'theory of Cognitive development'.
Hyperopia	Hyperopia, also known as farsightedness, longsightedness or hypermetropia, is a defect of vision caused by an imperfection in the eye (often when the eyeball is too short or when the lens cannot become round enough), causing difficulty focusing on near objects, and in extreme cases causing a sufferer to be unable to focus on objects at any distance. As an object moves toward the eye, the eye must increase its power to keep the image in focus on the retina. If the power of the cornea and lens is insufficient, as in Hyperopia, the image will appear blurred.
Otitis media	Otitis media is inflammation of the middle ear, or middle ear infection. Otitis media occurs in the area between the ear drum and the inner ear, including a duct known as the eustachian tube. It is one of the two categories of ear inflammation that can underlie what is commonly called an earache, the other being otitis externa.
Smoking	Smoking is a practice in which a substance, most commonly tobacco, is burned and the smoke tasted or inhaled. This is primarily practised as a route of administration for recreational drug use, as combustion releases the active substances in drugs such as nicotine and makes them available for absorption through the lungs.

Chapter 20. School-Age Child,

Health promotion	Health promotion has been defined by the World Health Organization's 2005 Bangkok Charter for Health promotion in a Globalized World as 'the process of enabling people to increase control over their health and its determinants, and thereby improve their health'. The primary means of Health promotion occur through developing healthy public policy that addresses the prerequisities of health such as income, housing, food security, employment, and quality working conditions. There is a tendency among public health officials and governments -- and this is especially the case in liberal nations such as Canada and the USA -- to reduce Health promotion to health education and social marketing focused on changing behavioral risk factors.
Kinesthetic learning	Kinesthetic learning is a learning style in which learning takes place by the student actually carrying out a physical activity, rather than listening to a lecture or merely watching a demonstration. It is also referred to as tactile learning. People with a kinesthetic learning style are also commonly known as do-ers.
Auditory	Auditory means of or relating to the process of hearing: · Auditory system, the neurological structures and pathways of sound perception. · Sound, the physical signal perceived by the Auditory system. · Hearing (sense), is the Auditory sense, the sense by which sound is perceived. · Ear, the Auditory end organ. · Cochlea, the Auditory branch of the inner ear. · Auditory illusion, sound trick analogous to an optical illusion. · Primary Auditory cortex, the part of the higher-level of the brain that serves hearing. · External Auditory meatus, the ear canal · Auditory scene analysis, the process by which a scene containing many sounds is perceived · Auditory phonetics, the science of the sounds of language · Auditory imagery, hearing in head in the absence of sound
Auditory learning	Auditory learning is a learning style in which a person learns through listening. An auditory learner depends on hearing and speaking as a main way of learning. Auditory learners must be able to hear what is being said in order to understand and may have difficulty with instructions that are written.
Language development	Language development is a process starting early in human life, when a person begins to acquire language by learning it as it is spoken and by mimicry. Children's language development moves from simple to complex. Infants start without language.
Case study	A Case study is a research methodology common in social science. It is based on an in-depth investigation of a single individual, group, or event to explore causation in order to find underlying principles.
Learning disability	Learning disability is a classification including several disorders in which a person has difficulty learning in a typical manner, usually caused by an unknown factor or factors. The unknown factor is the disorder that affects the brain's ability to receive and process information.

Individuals with Disabilities Education Act	The Individuals with Disabilities Education Act is a United States federal law that governs how states and public agencies provide early intervention, special education, and related services to children with disabilities. It addresses the educational needs of children with disabilities from birth to age 18 or 21 in cases that involve 13 specified categories of disability. The IDEA is 'spending clause' legislation, meaning that it only applies to those States and their local educational agencies that accept federal funding under the IDEA. While States declining such funding are not subject to the IDEA, all States have accepted funding under this statute and are subject to it.
Human development	Human development is the process of growing to maturity. In biological terms, this entails growth from a one-celled zygote to an adult human being. Development begins with fertilization, the process by which the male gamete, the sperm cell, and the female gamete, the egg, fuse to produce a zygote.
Cardiovascular disease	Cardiovascular disease or Cardiovascular diseases refers to the class of diseases that involve the heart or blood vessels (arteries and veins). While the term technically refers to any disease that affects the cardiovascular system (as used in MeSH), it is usually used to refer to those related to atherosclerosis (arterial disease). These conditions have similar causes, mechanisms, and treatments.
Child abuse	Child abuse is the physical or psychological/emotional mistreatment of children. In the United States, the Centers for Disease Control and Prevention (CDC) define child maltreatment as any act or series of acts of commission or omission by a parent or other caregiver that results in harm, potential for harm, or threat of harm to a child. Most Child abuse occurs in a child's home, with a smaller amount occurring in the organizations, schools or communities the child interacts with.
Risk factor	A Risk factor is a variable associated with an increased risk of disease or infection. Risk factors are correlational and not necessarily causal, because correlation does not imply causation. For example, being young cannot be said to cause measles, but young people are more at risk as they are less likely to have developed immunity during a previous epidemic.
Sex education	Sex education is a broad term used to describe education about human sexual anatomy, sexual reproduction, sexual intercourse, reproductive health, emotional relations, reproductive rights and responsibilities, abstinence, contraception, and other aspects of human sexual behavior. Common avenues for sex education are parents or caregivers, school programs, and public health campaigns. Overview

Chapter 20. School-Age Child,

Sexual function	Sexual function is a model developed at the Karolinska Institute in Stockholm, Sweden, defining different aspects of the assessment of sexual dysfunction comprises the following components. Firstly, relevant aspects of sexual function are defined on the basis of a modified version of Masters and Johnson's pioneer work. The aspects of sexual function defined as being relevant to the assessment include sexual desire, erection, orgasm and ejaculation.
Child depression	Child depression is a mental illness in which a child feels worthless and is generally sad for a long time each day. About 5 percent of children and adolescents suffer from depression at any given time. Child depression can occur in both small children and teens.
Symptom	A symptom is a departure from normal function or feeling which is noticed by a patient, indicating the presence of disease or abnormality. A symptom is subjective, observed by the patient, and not measured. A symptom may not be a malady, for example symptoms of pregnancy.
Alcohol abuse	Alcohol abuse, as described in the DSM-IV, is a psychiatric diagnosis describing the recurring use of alcoholic beverages despite negative consequences. It is differentiated from alcohol dependence by the lack of symptoms such as tolerance and withdrawal. Alcohol abuse is sometimes referred to by the less specific term alcoholism.
Seat belt	A Seat belt, sometimes called a safety belt, is a safety harness designed to secure the occupant of a vehicle against harmful movement that may result from a collision or a sudden stop. As part of an overall automobile passive safety system, Seat belts are intended to reduce injuries by stopping the wearer from hitting hard interior elements of the vehicle, or other passengers (the so-called second impact), are in the correct position for the airbag to deploy and prevent the passenger from being thrown from the vehicle. Seat belts also absorb energy by being designed to stretch during an impact, so that there is less speed differential between the passenger's body and their vehicle interior, and also to spread the loading of impact on the passengers body.
Hepatitis B	Hepatitis B is an infectious illness caused by hepatitis B virus (HBV) which infects the liver of hominoidea, including humans, and causes an inflammation called hepatitis. Originally known as 'serum hepatitis', the disease has caused epidemics in parts of Asia and Africa, and it is endemic in China. About a third of the world's population, more than 2 billion people, have been infected with the hepatitis B virus.

Prescription drug	A Prescription drug is a licensed medicine that is regulated by legislation to require a prescription before it can be obtained. The term is used to distinguish it from over-the-counter drugs which can be obtained without a prescription. Different jurisdictions have different definitions of what constitutes a Prescription drug.
Immunization	Immunization is the process by which an individual's immune system becomes fortified against an agent (known as the immunogen). When an immune system is exposed to molecules that are foreign to the body (non-self), it will orchestrate an immune response, but it can also develop the ability to quickly respond to a subsequent encounter (through immunological memory). This is a function of the adaptive immune system.
Vaccination	Vaccination is the administration of antigenic material (the vaccine) to produce immunity to a disease. Vaccines can prevent or ameliorate the effects of infection by many pathogens. There is strong evidence for the influenza vaccine, the HPV vaccine and the chicken pox vaccine among others.
Vaccine	A vaccine is a biological preparation that improves immunity to a particular disease. A vaccine typically contains an agent that resembles a disease-causing microorganism, and is often made from weakened or killed forms of the microbe or its toxins. The agent stimulates the body's immune system to recognize the agent as foreign, destroy it, and 'remember' it, so that the immune system can more easily recognize and destroy any of these microorganisms that it later encounters.
Cancer	Cancer (medical term: malignant neoplasm) is a class of diseases in which a group of cells display uncontrolled growth, invasion that intrudes upon and destroys adjacent tissues, and sometimes metastasis, or spreading to other locations in the body via lymph or blood. These three malignant properties of cancers differentiate them from benign tumors, which do not invade or metastasize. Researchers divide the causes of cancer into two groups: those with an environmental cause and those with a hereditary genetic cause.
Data collection	Data collection is a term used to describe a process of preparing and collecting data - for example as part of a process improvement or similar project. The purpose of Data collection is to obtain information to keep on record, to make decisions about important issues, to pass information on to others. Primarily, data is collected to provide information regarding a specific topic.

Chapter 20. School-Age Child,

Data collection usually takes place early on in an improvement project, and is often formalised through a Data collection plan which often contains the following activity.

· Pre collection activity - Agree goals, target data, definitions, methods· Collection - Data collection· Present Findings - usually involves some form of sorting analysis and/or presentation.

Health care	Health care , refers to the treatment and management of illness, and the preservation of health through services offered by the medical, dental, complementary and alternative medicine, pharmaceutical, clinical laboratory sciences , nursing, and allied health professions. Health care embraces all the goods and services designed to promote health, including 'preventive, curative and palliative interventions, whether directed to individuals or to populations'. Before the term Health care became popular, English-speakers referred to medicine or to the health sector and spoke of the treatment and prevention of illness and disease.
Health education	Health education is the profession of educating people about health. Areas within this profession encompass environmental health, physical health, social health, emotional health, intellectual health, and spiritual health. It can be defined as the principle by which individuals and groups of people learn to behave in a manner conducive to the promotion, maintenance, or restoration of health.

1. _____ is a term used to describe a process of preparing and collecting data - for example as part of a process improvement or similar project. The purpose of _____ is to obtain information to keep on record, to make decisions about important issues, to pass information on to others. Primarily, data is collected to provide information regarding a specific topic.

   _____ usually takes place early on in an improvement project, and is often formalised through a _____ plan which often contains the following activity.

   · Pre collection activity - Agree goals, target data, definitions, methods· Collection - _____ · Present Findings - usually involves some form of sorting analysis and/or presentation.

   a. Bacteriophage
   b. Data collection
   c. Basal-like carcinoma
   d. Bladder cancer

2. . A _____ is a variable associated with an increased risk of disease or infection.

Chapter 20. School-Age Child,

_____s are correlational and not necessarily causal, because correlation does not imply causation. For example, being young cannot be said to cause measles, but young people are more at risk as they are less likely to have developed immunity during a previous epidemic.

    a. Years of potential life lost
    b. Risk factor
    c. Late effect
    d. Bacteriophage

3.   _____ is a sleep disorder characterized by pauses in breathing during sleep. Each episode, called an apnea , from α- (a-), privative, πνÎειν (pnéein), to breathe), lasts long enough so that one or more breaths are missed, and such episodes occur repeatedly throughout sleep. The standard definition of any apneic event includes a minimum 10 second interval between breaths, with either a neurological arousal (a 3-second or greater shift in EEG frequency, measured at C3, C4, O1, or O2), a blood oxygen desaturation of 3-4% or greater, or both arousal and desaturation.

    a. Dyspnea
    b. Bacteriophage
    c. Baroreflex
    d. Sleep apnea

4.   An _____ is a system of biological structures and processes within an organism that protects against disease by identifying and killing pathogens and tumour cells. It detects a wide variety of agents, from viruses to parasitic worms, and needs to distinguish them from the organism's own healthy cells and tissues in order to function properly. Detection is complicated as pathogens can evolve rapidly, producing adaptations that avoid the _____ and allow the pathogens to successfully infect their hosts.

    a. Allergy
    b. Immune system
    c. Antigen
    d. Immunoglobulin A

5.   A _____ is an organ system that gives animals (including humans) the ability to move using the muscular and skeletal systems. The _____ provides form, stability, and movement to the body.

It is made up of the body's bones (the skeleton), muscles, cartilage, tendons, ligaments, joints, and other connective tissue (the tissue that supports and binds tissues and organs together).

    a. Plantarflexion
    b. Musculoskeletal system
    c. Flexion
    d. Bacteriophage

1. b
2. b
3. d
4. b
5. b

You can take the complete Chapter Practice Test

for Chapter 20. School-Age Child,
on all key terms, persons, places, and concepts.

Online 99 Cents

http://www.epub1625.32.20273.20.cram101.com/

Use www.Cram101.com for all your study needs

including Cram101's online interactive problem solving labs in

chemistry, statistics, mathematics, and more.

Chapter 21. Adolescent,

_____ Adipose tissue

_____ Adrenal glands

_____ Cardiovascular system

_____ Gonadotropin-releasing hormone

_____ Luteinizing hormone

_____ Pituitary gland

_____ Acne

_____ Respiratory system

_____ Sebaceous gland

_____ Nocturnal emission

_____ Scoliosis

_____ Turner syndrome

_____ Risk factor

_____ Vitamin D

_____ Anorexia nervosa

_____ Bulimia nervosa

_____ Eating disorder

_____ Staphylococcus aureus

_____ Cognitive development

CHAPTER OUTLINE: KEY TERMS, PEOPLE, PLACES, CONCEPTS

	Language development
	Pregnancy
	Hepatitis B
	Herpes simplex
	Infectious mononucleosis
	Meningococcal disease
	Substance abuse
	Breast self-examination
	Cervical cancer
	Testicular cancer
	Cancer
	Vaccine
	Health care

Chapter 21. Adolescent,

Adipose tissue	In histology, Adipose tissue or body fat or just fat is loose connective tissue composed of adipocytes. It is technically composed of roughly only 80% fat; fat in its solitary state exists in the liver and muscles. Adipose tissue is derived from lipoblasts.
Adrenal glands	In mammals, the adrenal glands are the star-shaped endocrine glands that sit on top of the kidneys. They are chiefly responsible for releasing hormones in conjunction with stress through the synthesis of corticosteroids and catecholamines, including cortisol and adrenaline (epinephrine), respectively. Anatomically, the adrenal glands are located in the retroperitoneum situated atop the kidneys, one on each side.
Cardiovascular system	The circulatory system is an organ system that passes nutrients (such as amino acids and electrolytes), gases, hormones, blood cells, etc. to and from cells in the body to help fight diseases and help stabilize body temperature and pH to maintain homeostasis. This system may be seen strictly as a blood distribution network, but some consider the circulatory system as composed of the Cardiovascular system, which distributes blood, and the lymphatic system, which distributes lymph.
Gonadotropin-releasing hormone	Gonadotropin-releasing hormone is a tropic peptide hormone responsible for the release of FSH and LH from the anterior pituitary. GnRH is synthesized and released from neurons within the hypothalamus. The gene, GNRH1, for the GnRH precursor is located on chromosome 8. In mammals, the linear decapeptide end-product is synthesized from a 92-amino acid preprohormone in the preoptic anterior hypothalamus.
Luteinizing hormone	Luteinizing hormone is a hormone produced by the anterior pituitary gland. · In the female, an acute rise of Luteinizing hormone - the Luteinizing hormone surge - triggers ovulation and corpus luteum development. · In the male, where Luteinizing hormone had also been called Interstitial Cell Stimulating Hormone , it stimulates Leydig cell production of testosterone. Luteinizing hormone is a heterodimeric glycoprotein. Each monomeric unit is a glycoprotein molecule; one alpha and one beta subunit make the full, functional protein.
Pituitary gland	The pituitary gland, or hypophysis, is an endocrine gland about the size of a pea and weighing 0.5 g (0.02 oz).. It is a protrusion off the bottom of the hypothalamus at the base of the brain, and rests in a small, bony cavity (sella turcica) covered by a dural fold (diaphragma sellae).

Acne	Acne is a general term used for eruptive disease of the skin. It is sometimes used as a synonym for Acne vulgaris. However, there are several different types of Acne.
Respiratory system	The respiratory system's function is to allow gas exchange to all parts of the body. The space between the alveoli and the capillaries, the anatomy or structure of the exchange system, and the precise physiological uses of the exchanged gases vary depending on the organism. In humans and other mammals, for example, the anatomical features of the respiratory system include airways, lungs, and the respiratory muscles.
Sebaceous gland	The Sebaceous glands are microscopic glands in the skin which secrete an oily/waxy matter, called sebum, to lubricate the skin and hair of mammals. In humans, they are found in greatest abundance on the face and scalp, though they are distributed throughout all skin sites except the palms and soles. In the eyelids, meibomian Sebaceous glands secrete sebum into tears.
Nocturnal emission	A nocturnal emission involves either ejaculation during sleep for a male, or lubrication of the vagina for a female. It is also called a wet dream, and is sometimes considered a type of spontaneous orgasm. Nocturnal emissions are most common during adolescence and early young adult years.
Scoliosis	Scoliosis is a medical condition in which a person's spine is curved from side to side. Although it is a complex three-dimensional deformity, on an X-ray, viewed from the rear, the spine of an individual with scoliosis may look more like an 'S' or a 'C' than a straight line. Scoliosis is typically classified as either congenital (caused by vertebral anomalies present at birth), idiopathic (cause unknown, subclassified as infantile, juvenile, adolescent, or adult, according to when onset occurred), or neuromuscular (having developed as a secondary symptom of another condition, such as spina bifida, cerebral palsy, spinal muscular atrophy, or physical trauma Patients having reached skeletal maturity are less likely to have a worsening case.
Turner syndrome	Turner syndrome, of which monosomy X (absence of an entire sex chromosome, the Barr body) is most common. It is a chromosomal abnormality in which all or part of one of the sex chromosomes is absent (unaffected humans have 46 chromosomes, of which two are sex chromosomes). Typical females have two X chromosomes, but in Turner syndrome, one of those sex chromosomes is missing or has other abnormalities.
Risk factor	A Risk factor is a variable associated with an increased risk of disease or infection. Risk factors are correlational and not necessarily causal, because correlation does not imply causation.

Chapter 21. Adolescent,

Vitamin D	Vitamin D is a group of fat-soluble prohormones, the two major forms of which are Vitamin D_2 (or ergocalciferol) and Vitamin D_3 (or cholecalciferol). Vitamin D obtained from sun exposure, food, and supplements, is biologically inert and must undergo two hydroxylation reactions to be activated in the body. Calcitriol (1,25-Dihydroxycholecalciferol) is the active form of Vitamin D found in the body.
Anorexia nervosa	Anorexia nervosa is a psychiatric illness that describes an eating disorder characterized by extremely low body weight and body image distortion with an obsessive fear of gaining weight. Individuals with Anorexia nervosa are known to control body weight commonly through the means of voluntary starvation, excessive exercise, or other weight control measures such as diet pills or diuretic drugs. While the condition primarily affects adolescent females, approximately 10% of people with the diagnosis are male.
Bulimia nervosa	Bulimia nervosa is an eating disorder characterized by restraining of food intake for a period of time followed by an over intake or binging period that results in feelings of guilt and low self-esteem. The median age of onset is 18. Sufferers attempt to overcome these feelings in a number of ways. The most common form is defensive vomiting, sometimes called purging; fasting, the use of laxatives, enemas, diuretics, and over exercising are also common.
Eating disorder	Eating disorders refer to a group of conditions characterized by abnormal eating habits that may involve either insufficient or excessive food intake to the detriment of an individual's physical and mental health. bulimia nervosa, anorexia nervosa being the most common specific forms in the United States. Though primarily thought of as affecting females (an estimated 5-10 million being affected in the U.S)., eating disorders affect males as well (an estimated 1 million U.S. males being affected).
Staphylococcus aureus	Staphylococcus aureus is a facultatively anaerobic, gram positive coccus and is the most common cause of staph infections. It is a spherical bacterium, frequently part of the skin flora found in the nose and on skin. About 20% of the population are long-term carriers of S. aureus.
Cognitive development	Cognitive development is a field of study in neuroscience and psychology focusing on a child's development in terms of information processing, conceptual resources, perceptual skill, language learning, and other aspects of brain development and cognitive psychology. A large portion of research has gone into understanding how a child conceptualizes the world. Jean Piaget was a major force in the founding of this field, forming his 'theory of Cognitive development'.
Language development	Language development is a process starting early in human life, when a person begins to acquire language by learning it as it is spoken and by mimicry. Children's language development moves from simple to complex. Infants start without language.

Pregnancy	Pregnancy is the carrying of one or more offspring, known as a fetus or embryo, inside the womb of a female. In a pregnancy, there can be multiple gestations, as in the case of twins or triplets. Human pregnancy is the most studied of all mammalian pregnancies.
Hepatitis B	Hepatitis B is an infectious illness caused by hepatitis B virus (HBV) which infects the liver of hominoidea, including humans, and causes an inflammation called hepatitis. Originally known as 'serum hepatitis', the disease has caused epidemics in parts of Asia and Africa, and it is endemic in China. About a third of the world's population, more than 2 billion people, have been infected with the hepatitis B virus.
Herpes simplex	Herpes simplex is a viral disease caused by both herpes simplex virus type 1 (HSV-1) and type 2 (HSV-2). Infection with the herpes virus is categorized into one of several distinct disorders based on the site of infection. Oral herpes, the visible symptoms of which are colloquially called cold sores or fever blisters, infects the face and mouth.
Infectious mononucleosis	Infectious mononucleosis is an infectious, widespread viral disease caused by the Epstein-Barr virus (EBV), one type of herpes virus, to which more than 90% of adults have been exposed. It's not chronic. Most people are exposed to the virus as children, when the disease produces no noticeable symptoms or only flu-like symptoms.
Meningococcal disease	Meningococcal disease describes infections caused by the bacterium Neisseria meningitidis (also termed meningococcus). It carries a high mortality rate if untreated. While best known as a cause of meningitis, widespread blood infection (sepsis) is more damaging and dangerous.
Substance abuse	Substance abuse also known as drug abuse, refers to a maladaptive pattern of use of a substance that is not considered dependent. The term 'drug abuse' does not exclude dependency, but is otherwise used in a similar manner in nonmedical contexts. The terms have a huge range of definitions related to taking a psychoactive drug or performance enhancing drug for a non-therapeutic or non-medical effect.
Breast self-examination	Breast self-examination (Breast self-examinationE) is a method of finding abnormalities of the breast, for early detection of breast cancer. The method involves the woman herself looking at and feeling each breast for possible lumps, distortions or swelling. Breast self-examinationE was once promoted heavily as a means of finding cancer at a more curable stage, but randomized controlled studies found that it was not effective in preventing death, and actually caused harm through needless biopsies and surgery.
Cervical cancer	Cervical cancer is malignant neoplasm of the cervix uteri or cervical area. It may present with vaginal bleeding, but symptoms may be absent until the cancer is in its advanced stages.

Chapter 21. Adolescent,

Testicular cancer	Testicular cancer is cancer that develops in the testicles, a part of the male reproductive system. In the United States, between 7,500 and 8,000 diagnoses of testicular cancer are made each year. Over his lifetime, a man's risk of testicular cancer is roughly 1 in 250 (0.4%).
Cancer	Cancer (medical term: malignant neoplasm) is a class of diseases in which a group of cells display uncontrolled growth, invasion that intrudes upon and destroys adjacent tissues, and sometimes metastasis, or spreading to other locations in the body via lymph or blood. These three malignant properties of cancers differentiate them from benign tumors, which do not invade or metastasize. Researchers divide the causes of cancer into two groups: those with an environmental cause and those with a hereditary genetic cause.
Vaccine	A vaccine is a biological preparation that improves immunity to a particular disease. A vaccine typically contains an agent that resembles a disease-causing microorganism, and is often made from weakened or killed forms of the microbe or its toxins. The agent stimulates the body's immune system to recognize the agent as foreign, destroy it, and 'remember' it, so that the immune system can more easily recognize and destroy any of these microorganisms that it later encounters.
Health care	Health care , refers to the treatment and management of illness, and the preservation of health through services offered by the medical, dental, complementary and alternative medicine, pharmaceutical, clinical laboratory sciences , nursing, and allied health professions. Health care embraces all the goods and services designed to promote health, including 'preventive, curative and palliative interventions, whether directed to individuals or to populations'. Before the term Health care became popular, English-speakers referred to medicine or to the health sector and spoke of the treatment and prevention of illness and disease.

Chapter 21. Adolescent,

1. A _____ involves either ejaculation during sleep for a male, or lubrication of the vagina for a female. It is also called a wet dream, and is sometimes considered a type of spontaneous orgasm.

   _____s are most common during adolescence and early young adult years.

   a. Polyphasic sleep
   b. Polysomnographic technician
   c. Power nap
   d. Nocturnal emission

2. A _____ is a variable associated with an increased risk of disease or infection. _____s are correlational and not necessarily causal, because correlation does not imply causation. For example, being young cannot be said to cause measles, but young people are more at risk as they are less likely to have developed immunity during a previous epidemic.

   a. Years of potential life lost
   b. Disease surveillance
   c. Late effect
   d. Risk factor

3. In mammals, the _____ are the star-shaped endocrine glands that sit on top of the kidneys. They are chiefly responsible for releasing hormones in conjunction with stress through the synthesis of corticosteroids and catecholamines, including cortisol and adrenaline (epinephrine), respectively.

   Anatomically, the _____ are located in the retroperitoneum situated atop the kidneys, one on each side.

   a. Adrenal glands
   b. ovaries
   c. abdominal exam
   d. Achilles tendon

4. _____ is an infectious, widespread viral disease caused by the Epstein-Barr virus (EBV), one type of herpes virus, to which more than 90% of adults have been exposed. It's not chronic. Most people are exposed to the virus as children, when the disease produces no noticeable symptoms or only flu-like symptoms.

   a. Infectious pancreatic necrosis
   b. Orthohepadnavirus
   c. Infectious mononucleosis
   d. Andes virus

5. . In histology, _____ or body fat or just fat is loose connective tissue composed of adipocytes. It is technically composed of roughly only 80% fat; fat in its solitary state exists in the liver and muscles. _____ is derived from lipoblasts.

   a. Adipose tissue

b. Achilles tendon

c. Acute HIV infection

d. Adenoviridae

1. d
2. d
3. a
4. c
5. a

You can take the complete Chapter Practice Test

for Chapter 21. Adolescent,
on all key terms, persons, places, and concepts.

Online 99 Cents

http://www.epub1625.32.20273.21.cram101.com/

Use www.Cram101.com for all your study needs

including Cram101's online interactive problem solving labs in

chemistry, statistics, mathematics, and more.

CHAPTER OUTLINE: KEY TERMS, PEOPLE, PLACES, CONCEPTS

Adrenocorticotropic hormone

Risk factor

Cardiovascular disease

Life expectancy

Maternal death

Health care

Physical examination

Blood pressure

Health promotion

Congenital rubella syndrome

Hepatitis B

Lyme disease

Metabolic syndrome

Cervical cancer

Genital herpes

Meningococcal disease

Vaccine

Weight gain

Iron deficiency

	Health effect
	Cognitive development
	Alcohol abuse
	Epididymitis
	Infertility
	Oral health
	Prenatal care
	Genetic counseling
	Genetic testing
	Noise pollution
	Case study
	Prenatal diagnosis
	Carbon monoxide
	Data collection
	Prescription drug
	Weight loss

Adrenocorticotropic hormone	Adrenocorticotropic hormone is a polypeptide tropic hormone produced and secreted by the anterior pituitary gland. It is an important component of the hypothalamic-pituitary-adrenal axis and is often produced in response to biological stress . Its principal effects are increased production of corticosteroids and, as its name suggests, cortisol from the adrenal cortex.
Risk factor	A Risk factor is a variable associated with an increased risk of disease or infection. Risk factors are correlational and not necessarily causal, because correlation does not imply causation. For example, being young cannot be said to cause measles, but young people are more at risk as they are less likely to have developed immunity during a previous epidemic.
Cardiovascular disease	Cardiovascular disease or Cardiovascular diseases refers to the class of diseases that involve the heart or blood vessels (arteries and veins). While the term technically refers to any disease that affects the cardiovascular system (as used in MeSH), it is usually used to refer to those related to atherosclerosis (arterial disease). These conditions have similar causes, mechanisms, and treatments.
Life expectancy	Life expectancy is the average number of years of life remaining at a given age. The term is most often used in the human context, but used also in plant or animal ecology and the calculation is based on the analysis of life tables (also known as actuarial tables). The term may also be used in the context of manufactured objects although the related term shelf life is used for consumer products and the term mean time to breakdown (MTTB) is used in engineering literature.
Maternal death	Maternal death also 'obstetrical death' is the death of a woman during or shortly after a pregnancy. In 2000, the United Nations estimated global maternal mortality at 529,000, of which less than 1% occurred in the developed world. However, most of these deaths have been medically preventable for decades, because treatments to avoid such deaths have been well known since the 1950s.
Health care	Health care , refers to the treatment and management of illness, and the preservation of health through services offered by the medical, dental, complementary and alternative medicine, pharmaceutical, clinical laboratory sciences , nursing, and allied health professions. Health care embraces all the goods and services designed to promote health, including 'preventive, curative and palliative interventions, whether directed to individuals or to populations'. Before the term Health care became popular, English-speakers referred to medicine or to the health sector and spoke of the treatment and prevention of illness and disease.
Physical examination	Physical examination or clinical examination is the process by which a doctor investigates the body of a patient for signs of disease. It generally follows the taking of the medical history -- an account of the symptoms as experienced by the patient.

Chapter 22. Young Adult,

Blood pressure	Blood pressure is the pressure (force per unit area) exerted by circulating blood on the walls of blood vessels, and constitutes one of the principal vital signs. The pressure of the circulating blood decreases as it moves away from the heart through arteries and capillaries, and toward the heart through veins. When unqualified, the term Blood pressure usually refers to brachial arterial pressure: that is, in the major blood vessel of the upper left or right arm that takes blood away from the heart.
Health promotion	Health promotion has been defined by the World Health Organization's 2005 Bangkok Charter for Health promotion in a Globalized World as 'the process of enabling people to increase control over their health and its determinants, and thereby improve their health'. The primary means of Health promotion occur through developing healthy public policy that addresses the prerequisities of health such as income, housing, food security, employment, and quality working conditions. There is a tendency among public health officials and governments -- and this is especially the case in liberal nations such as Canada and the USA -- to reduce Health promotion to health education and social marketing focused on changing behavioral risk factors.
Congenital rubella syndrome	Congenital rubella syndrome can occur in a developing fetus of a pregnant woman who has contracted rubella during her first trimester. If infection occurs 0-28 days before conception, there is a 43% chance the infant will be affected. If the infection occurs 0-12 weeks after conception, there is a 51% chance the infant will be affected.
Hepatitis B	Hepatitis B is an infectious illness caused by hepatitis B virus (HBV) which infects the liver of hominoidea, including humans, and causes an inflammation called hepatitis. Originally known as 'serum hepatitis', the disease has caused epidemics in parts of Asia and Africa, and it is endemic in China. About a third of the world's population, more than 2 billion people, have been infected with the hepatitis B virus.
Lyme disease	Lyme disease, is an emerging infectious disease caused by at least three species of bacteria belonging to the genus Borrelia. Borrelia burgdorferi sensu stricto is the main cause of Lyme disease in the United States, whereas Borrelia afzelii and Borrelia garinii cause most European cases. The disease is named after the town of Lyme, Connecticut, USA, where a number of cases were identified in 1975. Although Allen Steere realized in 1978 that Lyme disease was a tick-borne disease, the cause of the disease remained a mystery until 1981, when B. burgdorferi was identified by Willy Burgdorfer.
Metabolic syndrome	Metabolic syndrome is a combination of medical disorders that, when occurring together, increase the risk of developing cardiovascular disease and diabetes. It affects one in five people in the United States and prevalence increases with age. Some studies have shown the prevalence in the USA to be an estimated 25% of the population.
Cervical cancer	Cervical cancer is malignant neoplasm of the cervix uteri or cervical area.

It may present with vaginal bleeding, but symptoms may be absent until the cancer is in its advanced stages. Treatment consists of surgery (including local excision) in early stages and chemotherapy and radiotherapy in advanced stages of the disease.

Genital herpes	Genital herpes refers to a genital infection by herpes simplex virus.

Following the classification HSV into two distinct categories of HSV-1 and HSV-2 in the 1960s, it was established that 'HSV-2 was below the waist, HSV-1 was above the waist'. Although Genital herpes is largely believed to be caused by HSV-2, genital HSV-1 infections are increasing and now exceed 50% in certain populations, and that rule of thumb no longer applies.

Meningococcal disease	Meningococcal disease describes infections caused by the bacterium Neisseria meningitidis (also termed meningococcus). It carries a high mortality rate if untreated. While best known as a cause of meningitis, widespread blood infection (sepsis) is more damaging and dangerous.

Vaccine	A vaccine is a biological preparation that improves immunity to a particular disease. A vaccine typically contains an agent that resembles a disease-causing microorganism, and is often made from weakened or killed forms of the microbe or its toxins. The agent stimulates the body's immune system to recognize the agent as foreign, destroy it, and 'remember' it, so that the immune system can more easily recognize and destroy any of these microorganisms that it later encounters.

Weight gain	Weight gain is an increase in body weight. This can be either an increase in muscle mass, fat deposits, or excess fluids such as water.

Description

Muscle gain or weight gain can occur as a result of exercise or bodybuilding, in which muscle size is increased through strength training.

Iron deficiency	Iron deficiency is one of the most commonly known forms of nutritional deficiencies. In the human body, iron is present in all cells and has several vital functions--as a carrier of oxygen to the tissues from the lungs in the form of hemoglobin, as a transport medium for electrons within the cells in the form of cytochromes, and as an integral part of enzyme reactions in various tissues. Too little iron can interfere with these vital functions and lead to morbidity and mortality.

Health effect	Health effects are changes in health resulting from exposure to a source. Health effects are an important consideration in many areas, such as hygiene, pollution studies, workplace safety, nutrition and health sciences in general. Some of the major environmental sources of Health effects are air pollution, water pollution, soil contamination, noise pollution and over-illumination.

Chapter 22. Young Adult,

Cognitive development	Cognitive development is a field of study in neuroscience and psychology focusing on a child's development in terms of information processing, conceptual resources, perceptual skill, language learning, and other aspects of brain development and cognitive psychology. A large portion of research has gone into understanding how a child conceptualizes the world. Jean Piaget was a major force in the founding of this field, forming his 'theory of Cognitive development'.
Alcohol abuse	Alcohol abuse, as described in the DSM-IV, is a psychiatric diagnosis describing the recurring use of alcoholic beverages despite negative consequences. It is differentiated from alcohol dependence by the lack of symptoms such as tolerance and withdrawal. Alcohol abuse is sometimes referred to by the less specific term alcoholism.
Epididymitis	Epididymitis is a medical condition in which there is inflammation of the epididymis (a curved structure at the back of the testicle in which sperm matures and is stored). This condition may be mildly to very painful, and the scrotum (sac containing the testicles) may become red, warm and swollen. It may be acute (of sudden onset) or rarely chronic.
Infertility	Infertility primarily refers to the biological inability of a person to contribute to conception. Infertility may also refer to the state of a woman who is unable to carry a pregnancy to full term. There are many biological causes of infertility, some which may be bypassed with medical intervention.
Oral health	Good oral health is the absence of disease, disorder, and injury from the mouth, especially from the teeth and gums. Dental pertains to the teeth, including dentistry. Topics related to the human mouth or teeth include: Contents: Top - 0-9 A B C D E F G H I J K L M N O P Q R S T U V W X Y Z Abfraction · Abrasion · Academy of General Dentistry · Accelerated Orthodontic Treatment · Acinic cell carcinoma · Acrodont · Adalbert J. Volck · Adenomatoid odontogenic tumor · Adhesive Dentistry · Aetna · Agar · Aggregatibacter actinomycetemcomitans · Aim toothpaste · Akers' clasp · Alberta Dental Association and College · Alfred Fones · Alfred P. Southwick · Alginic acid · Alice Timander · Allan G. Brodie · Alveolar bony defects · Alveolar osteitis · Alveolar process of maxilla · Alveolar ridge · Amalgam · Ameloblast · Ameloblastic fibroma · Ameloblastin · Ameloblastoma · Amelogenesis · Amelogenesis imperfecta · Amelogenin · American Academy of Cosmetic Dentistry · American Association of Endodontists · American Association of Orthodontists · American Dental Association · American Dental Education Association · American Dental Hygienists' Association · American Society of Dental Surgeons · American Student Dental Association · Amosan · Anbesol · Angular cheilitis · Anodontia · Anthony Hamilton-Smith, 3rd Baron Colwyn · Antoni CieszyÅ„ski · Apert syndrome · Apex locator · Aphthous ulcer · Applied kinesiology · Aquafresh · Archwire · Arizona Dental Association · Arm & Hammer · Armin Abron · Articaine · Articulator · Asian Journal of Oral and Maxillofacial Surgery

· Associazione Italiana Odontoiatri · Astring-O-Sol · Attrition · Australian Dental Association · Automatic toothpaste dispenser ·

Badri Teymourtash · Baltimore College of Dental Surgery · Barbed broach · Barry Cockcroft · Barodontalgia · Bartholomew Ruspini · Baylor College of Dentistry · Ben Harper · Ben Humble · Ben L. Salomon · Benign lymphoepithelial lesion · Bernard J. Cigrand · Bernard Nadler · Bessie Delany · Bill Allen · Bill Emmerson · Bill Osmanski · Billy Cannon · Bioactive glass · Biobloc · Biodontics · Black hairy tongue · BlanX · Bleeding on probing · Botryoid odontogenic cyst · Brachydont · Brachygnathism · Breath spray · Bridge · Bristol-Myers Squibb · British Dental Association · British Dental Health Foundation · British Dental Students' Association · British Orthodontic Society · British Society of Oral Implantology · Bruxism · Buccal mucosa · Buccal space ·

C. T. Mathew · CAD/CAM Dentistry · Calcifying epithelial odontogenic tumor · Calcifying odontogenic cyst · Calcium hydroxide · Calculus · California Dental Association · Canadian Academy of Endodontics · Canadian Association of Orthodontists · Canadian College of Dental Health · Canadian Dental Association · Canalicular adenoma · Canine tooth · Cantilever mechanics · Carbon dioxide laser · Caries vaccine · Carnassial · Case School of Dental Medicine · Cattle age determination · Cemento-osseous dysplasia · Cementoblast · Cementoblastoma · Cementoenamel junction · Cementogenesis · Cementum · Central giant cell granuloma · Central odontogenic fibroma · Central ossifying fibroma · Central Regional Dental Testing Service · Centric relation · Centro Escolar University · CEREC · Cervical loop · Chapin A. Harris · Chapped lips · Charles G. Maurice · Charles Goodall Lee · Charles H. Strub · Charles Murray Turpin · Charles Spence Bate · Charles Stent · Charlie Norwood · Cheilitis · Chen Hsing-yu · Chewable toothbrush · Chewiness · Chief Dental Officer · Chlorhexidine · Christian Medical and Dental Associations · Christian Medical and Dental Fellowship of Australia · Christian Medical and Dental Society · Church and Dwight · Cingulum · Cleft lip and palate · Colgate-Palmolive · Colgate · Commonly used terms of relationship and comparison in dentistry · Concrescence · Condensing osteitis · Configuration factor · Congenital epulis · Consultant Orthodontists Group · Consumers for Dental Choice · Cosmetic dentistry · Crest · Crispiness · Crossbite · Crouzon syndrome · Crown-to-root ratio · Crown · Crown · Crown lengthening · Crunchiness · Curve of spee · Cusp · Cusp of Carabelli ·

D. A. Pandu Memorial R. V. Dental College & Hospital, Bangalore · D.D.S. M.D. · Dan Crane · Darlie · David J. Acer · Deciduous · Deciduous teeth · Delta Dental · Dens evaginatus · Dens invaginatus · Dental-enamel junction · Dental Admission Test · Dental alveolus · Dental amalgam controversy · Dental anatomy · Dental anesthesia · Dental arches · Dental assistant · Dental auxiliary · Dental braces · Dental bur · Dental canaliculi · Dental caries · Dental college · Dental composite · Dental Council of India · Dental cyst · Dental dam · Dental disease · Dental drill · Dental emergency · Dental engine · Dental floss · Dental fluorosis · Dental follicle · Dental hygienist · Dental implant · Dental informatics · Dental instruments · Dental key

Chapter 22. Young Adult,

CHAPTER HIGHLIGHTS & NOTES: KEY TERMS, PEOPLE, PLACES, CONCEPTS

· Dental Laboratories Association · Dental laboratory · Dental lamina · Dental laser · Dental midline · Dental notation · Dental papilla · Dental pathology · Dental pellicle · Dental phobia · Dental plaque · Dental porcelain · Dental Practitioners' Association · Dental public health · Dental radiography · Dental restoration · Dental restorative materials · Dental sealant · Dental spa · Dental surgery · Dental syringe · Dental technician · Dental Technologists Association · Dental therapist · DenTek Oral Care · Dentifrice · Dentigerous Cyst · Dentin · Dentin dysplasia · Dentine bonding agents · Dentine hypersensitivity · Dentinogenesis · Dentinogenesis imperfecta · Dentistry · Dentistry Magazine · Dentistry throughout the world · Dentition · Dentrix · Dentures · Denturist · Desquamative gingivitis · Diane Legault · Diastema · Dilaceration · Doc Holliday · Don McLeroy · Donald Leake · Dr. Alban · Dr. Radley Tate · Dr. Tariq Faraj ·

E. Lloyd Du Brul · Eagle syndrome · Early childhood caries · Eastman Kodak · Ed Lafitte · Edentulism · Edward Angle · Edward Hudson · Edward Maynard · Egg tooth · Electric toothbrush · Elmex · Elsie Gerlach · Embrasure · Enamel cord · Enamel knot · Enamel lamellae · Enamel niche · Enamel organ · Enamel pearl · Enamel rod · Enamel spindles · Enamel tufts · Enamelin · Endodontic therapy · Endodontics · Epulis fissuratum · Er:YAG laser · Erosion · Eruption cyst · Erythroplakia · Euthymol · Ewald Fabian · Explorer · External resorption · Extraction ·

F. labii inferioris · Faculty of Dental Surgery · Faculty of General Dental Practice · False tooth · Fatima Jinnah Dental College · FDI World Dental Federation · FDI World Dental Federation notation · FDSRCS England · Felix Crawford · Fiberotomy · Filiform papilla · Fissured tongue · Fixed prosthodontics · Florida Dental Association · Fluoride therapy · Focal infection · Foliate papillae · Forensic dentistry · Frank Abbott · Frank Crowther · Frederick B. Moorehead · Frederick Bogue Noyes · Frederick J. Conboy · Free gingival margin · Frenulum linguae · Frey's syndrome · Fungiform papilla ·

G. Walter Dittmar · Gardner's syndrome · Gargling · Gaspard Fauteux · Gene Derricotte · General Dental Council · General Practice Residency · Geographic tongue · Georg Carabelli · George S. Long · Gerald Cardinale · Geriatric dentistry · Gerrit Wolsink · Giant cell fibroma · Gigantiform cementoma · Gingiva · Gingival and periodontal pockets · Gingival cyst of the adult · Gingival cyst of the newborn · Gingival enlargement · Gingival fibers · Gingival sulcus · Gingivectomy · Gingivitis · Giovanni Battista Orsenigo · Glandular odontogenic cyst · Glasgow Dental Hospital and School · Glass ionomer cement · GlaxoSmithKline · Gleem toothpaste · Glennon Engleman · Global Surgical · Globulomaxillary cyst · Glossitis · Glot-Up · Gnarled enamel · Gnathology · Gold teeth · Goldman School of Dental Medicine · Gomphosis · Göran Lindblad · Government Dental College, Bangalore · Granular cell tumor · Greene Vardiman Black · Gum graft · Gunadasa Amarasekara · Gustatory system ·

Halimeter · Halitosis · Hammaspeikko · Hard palate · Harold Albrecht · Harvard School of Dental Medicine · Head and neck anatomy · Healing of periapical lesions · Henry D. Cogswell

· Henry Schein · Henry Trendley Dean · Henryka Bartnicka-Tajchert · Hertwig's epithelial root sheath · Heterodont · Hexetidine · Horace Wells · Horse teeth · Hydrodynamic theory · Hyperdontia · Hypocone · Hypodontia · Hypoglossia · Hypsodont ·

I.P. Dental College · Ian Gainsford · Idiopathic osteosclerosis · Implant-supported bridge · Impression · Incisor · Inferior alveolar nerve · Inflammatory papillary hyperplasia · Ingestion · Inlays and onlays · Inner enamel epithelium · Integra lifesciences · Interdental brush · Interdental papilla · Interdental plate · Internal resorption · International Academy of Oral Medicine and Toxicology · International Association for Dental Research · International Christian Medical and Dental Association · Interrod enamel · Invisalign · Ipana · Isaac Schour ·

Jack Miller · James Garretson · James W. Holley, III · Jan Boubli · Jim Granberry · Jim Harrell, Jr.

Prenatal care	Prenatal care refers to the medical and nursing care recommended for women before and during pregnancy. The aim of good Prenatal care is to detect any potential problems early, to prevent them if possible (through recommendations on adequate nutrition, exercise, vitamin intake etc), and to direct the woman to appropriate specialists, hospitals, etc. if necessary.
Genetic counseling	Genetic counseling is the process by which patients or relatives, at risk of an inherited disorder, are advised of the consequences and nature of the disorder, the probability of developing or transmitting it, and the options open to them in management and family planning in order to prevent, avoid or ameliorate it. This complex process can be seen from diagnostic (the actual estimation of risk) and supportive aspects. A genetic counselor is a medical genetics expert with a master of science degree.
Genetic testing	Genetic testing allows the genetic diagnosis of vulnerabilities to inherit diseases, and can also be used to determine a child's paternity (genetic father) or a person's ancestry. Normally, every person carries two copies of every gene, one inherited from their mother, one inherited from their father. The human genome is believed to contain around 20,000 - 25,000 genes.
Noise pollution	Noise pollution is displeasing human-, animal- or machine-created sound that disrupts the activity or balance of human or animal life. The word noise comes from the Latin word nausea meaning seasickness. The source of most outdoor noise worldwide is transportation systems, including motor vehicle noise, aircraft noise and rail noise.
Case study	A Case study is a research methodology common in social science.

Chapter 22. Young Adult,

Prenatal diagnosis	Prenatal diagnosis or prenatal screening is testing for diseases or conditions in a fetus or embryo before it is born. The aim is to detect birth defects such as neural tube defects, Down syndrome, chromosome abnormalities, genetic diseases and other conditions, such as spina bifida, cleft palate, Tay Sachs disease, sickle cell anemia, thalassemia, cystic fibrosis, and fragile x syndrome. Screening can also be used for prenatal sex discernment.
Carbon monoxide	Carbon monoxide, with the chemical formula CO, is a colorless, odorless and tasteless, yet highly toxic gas. Its molecules consist of one carbon atom and one oxygen atom, connected by a covalent double bond and a dative covalent bond. It is the simplest oxocarbon, and can be viewed as the anhydride of formic acid (CH_2O_2).
Data collection	Data collection is a term used to describe a process of preparing and collecting data - for example as part of a process improvement or similar project. The purpose of Data collection is to obtain information to keep on record, to make decisions about important issues, to pass information on to others. Primarily, data is collected to provide information regarding a specific topic.
	Data collection usually takes place early on in an improvement project, and is often formalised through a Data collection plan which often contains the following activity.
	· Pre collection activity - Agree goals, target data, definitions, methods· Collection - Data collection· Present Findings - usually involves some form of sorting analysis and/or presentation.
Prescription drug	A Prescription drug is a licensed medicine that is regulated by legislation to require a prescription before it can be obtained. The term is used to distinguish it from over-the-counter drugs which can be obtained without a prescription. Different jurisdictions have different definitions of what constitutes a Prescription drug.
Weight loss	Weight loss, in the context of medicine, health or physical fitness, is a reduction of the total body mass, due to a mean loss of fluid, body fat or adipose tissue and/or lean mass, namely bone mineral deposits, muscle, tendon and other connective tissue. It can occur unintentionally due to an underlying disease or can arise from a conscious effort to improve an actual or perceived overweight or obese state.
	Unintentional weight loss
	Unintentional weight loss occurs in many diseases and conditions, including some very serious diseases such as cancer, AIDS, and a variety of other diseases.

Chapter 22. Young Adult,

0

1. _____ is the process by which patients or relatives, at risk of an inherited disorder, are advised of the consequences and nature of the disorder, the probability of developing or transmitting it, and the options open to them in management and family planning in order to prevent, avoid or ameliorate it. This complex process can be seen from diagnostic (the actual estimation of risk) and supportive aspects.

A genetic counselor is a medical genetics expert with a master of science degree.

a. Chromatin
b. Fibrinogen
c. Prolactin
d. Genetic counseling

2. _____ is a polypeptide tropic hormone produced and secreted by the anterior pituitary gland. It is an important component of the hypothalamic-pituitary-adrenal axis and is often produced in response to biological stress . Its principal effects are increased production of corticosteroids and, as its name suggests, cortisol from the adrenal cortex.

a. Endorphin
b. Intrinsic factor
c. Atrial natriuretic peptide
d. Adrenocorticotropic hormone

3. _____ allows the genetic diagnosis of vulnerabilities to inherit diseases, and can also be used to determine a child's paternity (genetic father) or a person's ancestry. Normally, every person carries two copies of every gene, one inherited from their mother, one inherited from their father. The human genome is believed to contain around 20,000 - 25,000 genes.

a. Chromatin
b. Fibrinogen
c. Prolactin
d. Genetic testing

4. _____ is an infectious illness caused by _____ virus (HBV) which infects the liver of hominoidea, including humans, and causes an inflammation called hepatitis. Originally known as 'serum hepatitis', the disease has caused epidemics in parts of Asia and Africa, and it is endemic in China. About a third of the world's population, more than 2 billion people, have been infected with the _____ virus.

a. Hepatitis B
b. Bacterial vaginosis
c. Kaposi's sarcoma-associated herpesvirus
d. Pediculosis pubis

5. . A _____ is a licensed medicine that is regulated by legislation to require a prescription before it can be obtained. The term is used to distinguish it from over-the-counter drugs which can be obtained without a prescription. Different jurisdictions have different definitions of what constitutes a _____.

Chapter 22. Young Adult,

a. Body surface area

b. Prescription drug

c. Bacteriophage

d. Genome

1. d
2. d
3. d
4. a
5. b

You can take the complete Chapter Practice Test

for Chapter 22. Young Adult,
on all key terms, persons, places, and concepts.

Online 99 Cents

http://www.epub1625.32.20273.22.cram101.com/

Use www.Cram101.com for all your study needs

including Cram101's online interactive problem solving labs in

chemistry, statistics, mathematics, and more.

CHAPTER OUTLINE: KEY TERMS, PEOPLE, PLACES, CONCEPTS

Adrenocorticotropic hormone

Cardiac output

Cardiovascular system

Osteoarthritis

Musculoskeletal system

Myocardial infarction

Mortality rate

Menopause

Life expectancy

Risk factor

Health insurance

Cancer

Health disparities

Health promotion

Cardiovascular disease

Alcohol abuse

Liver disease

Vitamin D

Sodium

_____ | Dental caries

_____ | Prevention

_____ | Cognitive development

_____ | Diabetic retinopathy

_____ | Age related macular degeneration

_____ | Presbycusis

_____ | Presbyopia

_____ | Hormone therapy

_____ | Case study

_____ | Health care

_____ | Symptom

_____ | Transtheoretical model

_____ | Maternal death

_____ | Sexual dysfunction

_____ | Sexual function

_____ | Blood pressure

_____ | Noise pollution

_____ | Hepatitis A

_____ | Hepatitis B

Chapter 23. Middle-Age Adult,

| | Health administration |

| | Mental health |

| | Occupational Safety and Health Administration |

| | Health economics |

Adrenocorticotropic hormone	Adrenocorticotropic hormone is a polypeptide tropic hormone produced and secreted by the anterior pituitary gland. It is an important component of the hypothalamic-pituitary-adrenal axis and is often produced in response to biological stress . Its principal effects are increased production of corticosteroids and, as its name suggests, cortisol from the adrenal cortex.
Cardiac output	Cardiac output (Q) is the volume of blood being pumped by the heart, in particular by a ventricle in a minute. This is measured in dm^3 min^{-1} (1 dm^3 equals 1000 cm^3 or 1 litre). An average Cardiac output would be 5L.min^{-1} for a human male and 4.5L.min^{-1} for a female.
Cardiovascular system	The circulatory system is an organ system that passes nutrients (such as amino acids and electrolytes), gases, hormones, blood cells, etc. to and from cells in the body to help fight diseases and help stabilize body temperature and pH to maintain homeostasis. This system may be seen strictly as a blood distribution network, but some consider the circulatory system as composed of the Cardiovascular system, which distributes blood, and the lymphatic system, which distributes lymph.
Osteoarthritis	Osteoarthritis is a group of diseases and mechanical abnormalities involving degradation of joints, including articular cartilage and the subchondral bone next to it. Clinical manifestations of OA may include joint pain, tenderness, stiffness, creaking, locking of joints, and sometimes local inflammation. In OA, a variety of potential forces--hereditary, developmental, metabolic, and mechanical--may initiate processes leading to loss of cartilage -- a strong protein matrix that lubricates and cushions the joints.

Chapter 23. Middle-Age Adult,

Musculoskeletal system	A Musculoskeletal system is an organ system that gives animals (including humans) the ability to move using the muscular and skeletal systems. The Musculoskeletal system provides form, stability, and movement to the body. It is made up of the body's bones (the skeleton), muscles, cartilage, tendons, ligaments, joints, and other connective tissue (the tissue that supports and binds tissues and organs together).
Myocardial infarction	Myocardial infarction or acute myocardial infarction commonly known as a heart attack, results from the interruption of blood supply to a part of the heart, causing heart cells to die. This is most commonly due to occlusion (blockage) of a coronary artery following the rupture of a vulnerable atherosclerotic plaque, which is an unstable collection of lipids (cholesterol and fatty acids) and white blood cells (especially macrophages) in the wall of an artery. The resulting ischemia (restriction in blood supply) and ensuing oxygen shortage, if left untreated for a sufficient period of time, can cause damage or death (infarction) of heart muscle tissue (myocardium).
Mortality rate	Mortality rate is a measure of the number of deaths (in general,) in some population, scaled to the size of that population, per unit time. Mortality rate is typically expressed in units of deaths per 1000 individuals per year; thus, a Mortality rate of 9.5 in a population of 100,000 would mean 950 deaths per year in that entire population. It is distinct from morbidity rate, which refers to the number of individuals in poor health during a given time period (the prevalence rate) or the number who currently have that disease (the incidence rate), scaled to the size of the population.
Menopause	Menopause is the permanent cessation of reproductive fertility some time before the end of the natural lifespan. The term was originally used to describe this reproductive change in human females, where the end of fertility was traditionally indicated by the permanent stopping of menstruation or 'menses'. The word 'Menopause' literally means the 'end of monthly cycles' from the Greek words pausis and the word root men (month).
Life expectancy	Life expectancy is the average number of years of life remaining at a given age. The term is most often used in the human context, but used also in plant or animal ecology and the calculation is based on the analysis of life tables (also known as actuarial tables). The term may also be used in the context of manufactured objects although the related term shelf life is used for consumer products and the term mean time to breakdown (MTTB) is used in engineering literature.
Risk factor	A Risk factor is a variable associated with an increased risk of disease or infection. Risk factors are correlational and not necessarily causal, because correlation does not imply causation. For example, being young cannot be said to cause measles, but young people are more at risk as they are less likely to have developed immunity during a previous epidemic.
Health insurance	Health insurance is insurance that pays for medical expenses. It is sometimes used more broadly to include insurance covering disability or long-term nursing or custodial care needs.

Cancer	Cancer (medical term: malignant neoplasm) is a class of diseases in which a group of cells display uncontrolled growth, invasion that intrudes upon and destroys adjacent tissues, and sometimes metastasis, or spreading to other locations in the body via lymph or blood. These three malignant properties of cancers differentiate them from benign tumors, which do not invade or metastasize. Researchers divide the causes of cancer into two groups: those with an environmental cause and those with a hereditary genetic cause.
Health disparities	Health disparities refer to gaps in the quality of health and health care across racial, ethnic, sexual orientation and socioeconomic groups. The Health Resources and Services Administration defines Health disparities as 'population-specific differences in the presence of disease, health outcomes, or access to health care.' In the United States, Health disparities are well documented in minority populations such as African Americans, Native Americans, Asian Americans, and Latinos. When compared to whites, these minority groups have higher incidence of chronic diseases, higher mortality, and poorer health outcomes.
Health promotion	Health promotion has been defined by the World Health Organization's 2005 Bangkok Charter for Health promotion in a Globalized World as 'the process of enabling people to increase control over their health and its determinants, and thereby improve their health'. The primary means of Health promotion occur through developing healthy public policy that addresses the prerequisities of health such as income, housing, food security, employment, and quality working conditions. There is a tendency among public health officials and governments -- and this is especially the case in liberal nations such as Canada and the USA -- to reduce Health promotion to health education and social marketing focused on changing behavioral risk factors.
Cardiovascular disease	Cardiovascular disease or Cardiovascular diseases refers to the class of diseases that involve the heart or blood vessels (arteries and veins). While the term technically refers to any disease that affects the cardiovascular system (as used in MeSH), it is usually used to refer to those related to atherosclerosis (arterial disease). These conditions have similar causes, mechanisms, and treatments.
Alcohol abuse	Alcohol abuse, as described in the DSM-IV, is a psychiatric diagnosis describing the recurring use of alcoholic beverages despite negative consequences. It is differentiated from alcohol dependence by the lack of symptoms such as tolerance and withdrawal. Alcohol abuse is sometimes referred to by the less specific term alcoholism.
Liver disease	Liver disease is a broad term describing any single number of diseases affecting the liver. Many are accompanied by jaundice caused by increased levels of bilirubin in the system.

Chapter 23. Middle-Age Adult,

Vitamin D	Vitamin D is a group of fat-soluble prohormones, the two major forms of which are Vitamin D_2 (or ergocalciferol) and Vitamin D_3 (or cholecalciferol). Vitamin D obtained from sun exposure, food, and supplements, is biologically inert and must undergo two hydroxylation reactions to be activated in the body. Calcitriol (1,25-Dihydroxycholecalciferol) is the active form of Vitamin D found in the body.
Sodium	Sodium is a metallic element with a symbol Na and atomic number 11. It is a soft, silvery-white, highly reactive metal and is a member of the alkali metals within 'group 1' . It has only one stable isotope, ^{23}Na. Elemental Sodium was first isolated by Sir Humphry Davy in 1806 by passing an electric current through molten Sodium hydroxide.
Dental caries	Dental caries is a disease wherein bacterial processes damage hard tooth structure. These tissues progressively break down, producing dental cavities. Two groups of bacteria are responsible for initiating caries: Streptococcus mutans and Lactobacilli.
Prevention	Prevention refers to: · Preventive medicine · Hazard Prevention, the process of risk study and elimination and mitigation in emergency management · Risk Prevention · Risk management · Preventive maintenance · Crime Prevention · Prevention, an album by Scottish band De Rosa · Prevention a magazine about health in the United States · Prevent (company), a textile company from Slovenia
Cognitive development	Cognitive development is a field of study in neuroscience and psychology focusing on a child's development in terms of information processing, conceptual resources, perceptual skill, language learning, and other aspects of brain development and cognitive psychology. A large portion of research has gone into understanding how a child conceptualizes the world. Jean Piaget was a major force in the founding of this field, forming his 'theory of Cognitive development'.
Diabetic retinopathy	Diabetic retinopathy is retinopathy (damage to the retina) caused by complications of diabetes mellitus, which can eventually lead to blindness. It is an ocular manifestation of systemic disease which affects up to 80% of all patients who have had diabetes for 10 years or more. Despite these intimidating statistics, research indicates that at least 90% of these new cases could be reduced if there was proper and vigilant treatment and monitoring of the eyes.

Age related macular degeneration	Age related macular degeneration is a medical condition which usually affects older adults that results in a loss of vision in the center of the visual field (the macula) because of damage to the retina. It occurs in 'dry' and 'wet' forms. It is a major cause of visual impairment in older adults (>50 years).
Presbycusis	Presbycusis, is the cumulative effect of aging on hearing. Also known as presbyacusis, it is defined as a progressive bilateral symmetrical age-related sensorineural hearing loss. The hearing loss is most marked at higher frequencies.
Presbyopia	Presbyopia describes the condition where the eye exhibits a progressively diminished ability to focus on near objects with age. Presbyopia's exact mechanisms are not known with certainty; however, the research evidence most strongly supports a loss of elasticity of the crystalline lens, although changes in the lens's curvature from continual growth and loss of power of the ciliary muscles (the muscles that bend and straighten the lens) have also been postulated as its cause. Similar to grey hair and wrinkles, Presbyopia is a symptom caused by the natural course of aging; the direct translation of the condition's name is 'elder eye'.
Hormone therapy	Hormone therapy, or hormonal therapy is the use of hormones in medical treatment. Treatment with hormone antagonists may also referred to as hormonal therapy. Wikipedia has the following articles regarding this topic: · Hormonal therapy (oncology) for treatment of cancer · Hormone replacement therapy (menopause) connected to menopause · Testosterone replacement in males with low levels due to disease or aging · Hormone replacement therapy (female-to-male) in sex reassignment therapy for transmen · Hormone replacement therapy (male-to-female) in sex reassignment therapy for transwomen · Hormone therapy in Klinefelter's syndrome · Hormone therapy in Turner syndrome · Growth hormone treatment for growth hormone deficiency · Thyroid hormone replacement in hypothyroidism · Chemical castration of violent sex offenders
Case study	A Case study is a research methodology common in social science.

Chapter 23. Middle-Age Adult,

Health care	Health care , refers to the treatment and management of illness, and the preservation of health through services offered by the medical, dental, complementary and alternative medicine, pharmaceutical, clinical laboratory sciences , nursing, and allied health professions. Health care embraces all the goods and services designed to promote health, including 'preventive, curative and palliative interventions, whether directed to individuals or to populations'. Before the term Health care became popular, English-speakers referred to medicine or to the health sector and spoke of the treatment and prevention of illness and disease.
Symptom	A symptom is a departure from normal function or feeling which is noticed by a patient, indicating the presence of disease or abnormality. A symptom is subjective, observed by the patient, and not measured. A symptom may not be a malady, for example symptoms of pregnancy.
Transtheoretical model	The Transtheoretical model in health psychology is intended to explain or predict a person's success or failure in achieving a proposed behavior change, such as developing different habits. It attempts to answer why the change 'stuck' or alternatively why the change was not made. The Transtheoretical model is also known by the acronym 'TTranstheoretical model' and by the term 'stages of change model'.
Maternal death	Maternal death also 'obstetrical death' is the death of a woman during or shortly after a pregnancy. In 2000, the United Nations estimated global maternal mortality at 529,000, of which less than 1% occurred in the developed world. However, most of these deaths have been medically preventable for decades, because treatments to avoid such deaths have been well known since the 1950s.
Sexual dysfunction	Sexual dysfunction, including desire, arousal or orgasm. To maximize the benefits of medications and behavioural techniques in the management of sexual dysfunction it is important to have a comprehensive approach to the problem,A thorough sexual history and assessment of general health and other sexual problems (if any) are very important. Assessing (performance) anxiety, guilt (associated with masturbation in many South-Asian men), stress and worry are integral to the optimal management of sexual dysfunction.
Sexual function	Sexual function is a model developed at the Karolinska Institute in Stockholm, Sweden, defining different aspects of the assessment of sexual dysfunction comprises the following components.

Firstly, relevant aspects of sexual function are defined on the basis of a modified version of Masters and Johnson's pioneer work. The aspects of sexual function defined as being relevant to the assessment include sexual desire, erection, orgasm and ejaculation.

Blood pressure	Blood pressure is the pressure (force per unit area) exerted by circulating blood on the walls of blood vessels, and constitutes one of the principal vital signs. The pressure of the circulating blood decreases as it moves away from the heart through arteries and capillaries, and toward the heart through veins. When unqualified, the term Blood pressure usually refers to brachial arterial pressure: that is, in the major blood vessel of the upper left or right arm that takes blood away from the heart.
Noise pollution	Noise pollution is displeasing human-, animal- or machine-created sound that disrupts the activity or balance of human or animal life. The word noise comes from the Latin word nausea meaning seasickness. The source of most outdoor noise worldwide is transportation systems, including motor vehicle noise, aircraft noise and rail noise.
Hepatitis A	Hepatitis A is an acute infectious disease of the liver caused by the hepatitis A virus (HAV), which is transmitted person-to-person by ingestion of contaminated food or water or through direct contact with an infectious person. Tens of millions of individuals worldwide are estimated to become infected with HAV each year. The time between infection and the appearance of the symptoms (the incubation period) is between two and six weeks and the average incubation period is 28 days.
Hepatitis B	Hepatitis B is an infectious illness caused by hepatitis B virus (HBV) which infects the liver of hominoidea, including humans, and causes an inflammation called hepatitis. Originally known as 'serum hepatitis', the disease has caused epidemics in parts of Asia and Africa, and it is endemic in China. About a third of the world's population, more than 2 billion people, have been infected with the hepatitis B virus.
Health administration	Health administration or healthcare administration is the field relating to leadership, management, and administration of hospitals, hospital networks, and health care systems. Health care administrators are considered health care professionals. The discipline is known by many names, including health management, healthcare management, health systems management, health care systems management, and medical and health services management.

Chapter 23. Middle-Age Adult,

Mental health	Mental health is a term used to describe either a level of cognitive or emotional well-being or an absence of a mental disorder. From perspectives of the discipline of positive psychology or holism Mental health may include an individual's ability to enjoy life and procure a balance between life activities and efforts to achieve psychological resilience. The World Health Organization defines Mental health as 'a state of well-being in which the individual realizes his or her own abilities, can cope with the normal stresses of life, can work productively and fruitfully, and is able to make a contribution to his or her community'.
Occupational Safety and Health Administration	The United States Occupational Safety and Health Administration is an agency of the United States Department of Labor. It was created by Congress of the United States under the Occupational Safety and Health Act, signed by President Richard M Nixon, on December 29, 1970. Its mission is to prevent work-related injuries, illnesses, and occupational fatality by issuing and enforcing rules called standards for workplace safety and health. The agency is headed by a Deputy Assistant Secretary of Labor.
Health economics	Health economics is a branch of economics concerned with issues related to scarcity in the allocation of health and health care. For example, it is now clear that medical debt is the principle cause of bankruptcy in the United States. In broad terms, health economists study the functioning of the health care system and the private and social causes of health-affecting behaviors such as smoking.

CHAPTER QUIZ: KEY TERMS, PEOPLE, PLACES, CONCEPTS

1. _____, is the cumulative effect of aging on hearing. Also known as presbyacusis, it is defined as a progressive bilateral symmetrical age-related sensorineural hearing loss. The hearing loss is most marked at higher frequencies.

   a. Deafblindness
   b. Central hearing loss
   c. Conductive hearing loss
   d. Presbycusis

2. . The circulatory system is an organ system that passes nutrients (such as amino acids and electrolytes), gases, hormones, blood cells, etc. to and from cells in the body to help fight diseases and help stabilize body temperature and pH to maintain homeostasis. This system may be seen strictly as a blood distribution network, but some consider the circulatory system as composed of the _____, which distributes blood, and the lymphatic system, which distributes lymph.

   a. Cardiovascular system
   b. Right ventricle
   c. Systemic circulation

Chapter 23. Middle-Age Adult,

Visit Cram101.com for full Practice Exams

3. _____ is a polypeptide tropic hormone produced and secreted by the anterior pituitary gland. It is an important component of the hypothalamic-pituitary-adrenal axis and is often produced in response to biological stress . Its principal effects are increased production of corticosteroids and, as its name suggests, cortisol from the adrenal cortex.

    a. Endorphin
    b. Intrinsic factor
    c. Atrial natriuretic peptide
    d. Adrenocorticotropic hormone

4. _____ has been defined by the World Health Organization's 2005 Bangkok Charter for _____ in a Globalized World as 'the process of enabling people to increase control over their health and its determinants, and thereby improve their health'. The primary means of _____ occur through developing healthy public policy that addresses the prerequisities of health such as income, housing, food security, employment, and quality working conditions. There is a tendency among public health officials and governments -- and this is especially the case in liberal nations such as Canada and the USA -- to reduce _____ to health education and social marketing focused on changing behavioral risk factors.

    a. Bacteriophage
    b. Health promotion
    c. Black Report
    d. Haven Institute

5. The _____ in health psychology is intended to explain or predict a person's success or failure in achieving a proposed behavior change, such as developing different habits. It attempts to answer why the change 'stuck' or alternatively why the change was not made.

    The _____ is also known by the acronym 'TTranstheoretical model' and by the term 'stages of change model'.

    a. Transtheoretical model
    b. Tardive dyskinesia
    c. Target lesion
    d. Tetanic contraction

1. d
2. a
3. d
4. b
5. a

You can take the complete Chapter Practice Test

for Chapter 23. Middle-Age Adult,
on all key terms, persons, places, and concepts.

Online 99 Cents

http://www.epub1625.32.20273.23.cram101.com/

Use www.Cram101.com for all your study needs

including Cram101's online interactive problem solving labs in

chemistry, statistics, mathematics, and more.

Chapter 24. Older Adult,

_____ Health promotion

_____ Urge incontinence

_____ Respiratory tract

_____ Kegel exercise

_____ Lewy bodies

_____ Mild cognitive impairment

_____ Multi-infarct dementia

_____ Sleep disorder

_____ Tympanic membrane

_____ Risk factor

_____ Decubitus ulcers

_____ Life expectancy

_____ Case study

_____ Geriatric depression

_____ Geriatric Depression Scale

_____ Depression

_____ Euthanasia

_____ Osteoporosis

_____ Heat stroke

Prevention

Pneumococcal infection

Alcohol abuse

Prescription drug

Prostate cancer

Cancer

Cancer screening

Acute care

Palliative care

Home care

Continuing care

Health care

Health insurance

Chapter 24. Older Adult,

Health promotion	Health promotion has been defined by the World Health Organization's 2005 Bangkok Charter for Health promotion in a Globalized World as 'the process of enabling people to increase control over their health and its determinants, and thereby improve their health'. The primary means of Health promotion occur through developing healthy public policy that addresses the prerequisities of health such as income, housing, food security, employment, and quality working conditions. There is a tendency among public health officials and governments -- and this is especially the case in liberal nations such as Canada and the USA -- to reduce Health promotion to health education and social marketing focused on changing behavioral risk factors.
Urge incontinence	Urge incontinence is a form of urinary incontinence. Urge incontinence is involuntary loss of urine occurring for no apparent reason while suddenly feeling the need or urge to urinate. The most common cause of Urge incontinence is involuntary and inappropriate detrusor muscle contractions.
Respiratory tract	In humans the Respiratory tract is the part of the anatomy that has to do with the process of respiration. The Respiratory tract is divided into 3 segments: · Upper Respiratory tract: nose and nasal passages, paranasal sinuses, and throat or pharynx · Respiratory airways: voice box or larynx, trachea, bronchi, and bronchioles · Lungs: respiratory bronchioles, alveolar ducts, alveolar sacs, and alveoli The Respiratory tract is a common site for infections. Upper Respiratory tract infections are probably the most common infections in the world. Most of the Respiratory tract exists merely as a piping system for air to travel in the lungs; alveoli are the only part of the lung that exchanges oxygen and carbon dioxide with the blood.
Kegel exercise	A Kegel exercise consists of contracting and relaxing the muscles that form part of the pelvic floor (which some people now colloquially call the 'Kegel muscles'). Explanation The aim of Kegel exercises is to improve muscle tone by strengthening the pubococcygeus muscles of the pelvic floor.

Lewy bodies	Lewy bodies are abnormal aggregates of protein that develop inside nerve cells in Parkinson's disease (PD) and some other disorders. They are identified under the microscope when histology is performed on the brain. Lewy bodies appear as spherical masses that displace other cell components.
Mild cognitive impairment	Mild cognitive impairment is a diagnosis given to individuals who have cognitive impairments beyond that expected for their age and education, but that do not interfere significantly with their daily activities. It is considered to be the boundary or transitional stage between normal aging and dementia. Although Mild cognitive impairment can present with a variety of symptoms, when memory loss is the predominant symptom it is termed 'amnestic Mild cognitive impairment' and is frequently seen as a risk factor for Alzheimer's disease.
Multi-infarct dementia	Multi-infarct dementia, is one type of vascular dementia. Vascular dementia is the second most common form of dementia after Alzheimer's disease (AD) in older adults. Multi-infarct dementia is thought to be an irreversible form of dementia, and its onset is caused by a number of small strokes or sometimes, one large stroke.
Sleep disorder	A Sleep disorder is a medical disorder of the sleep patterns of a person or animal. Some Sleep disorders are serious enough to interfere with normal physical, mental and emotional functioning. A test commonly ordered for some Sleep disorders is the polysomnogram. The most common Sleep disorders include: · Primary insomnia: Chronic difficulty in falling asleep and/or maintaining sleep when no other cause is found for these symptoms. · Bruxism: Involuntarily grinding or clenching of the teeth while sleeping · Delayed sleep phase syndrome (DSPS): inability to awaken and fall asleep at socially acceptable times but no problem with sleep maintenance, a disorder of circadian rhythms. Other such disorders are advanced sleep phase syndrome (ASPS) and Non-24-hour sleep-wake syndrome (Non-24), both much less common than DSPS. · Hypopnea syndrome: Abnormally shallow breathing or slow respiratory rate while sleeping · Narcolepsy: Excessive daytime sleepiness (EDS) often culminating in falling asleep spontaneously but unwillingly at inappropriate times. · Cataplexy, a sudden weakness in the motor muscles that can result in collapse to the floor. · Night terror, Pavor nocturnus, sleep terror disorder: abrupt awakening from sleep with behavior consistent with terror · Parasomnias: Disruptive sleep-related events involving inappropriate actions during sleep stages - sleep walking and night-terrors are examples. · Periodic limb movement disorder (PLMD): Sudden involuntary movement of arms and/or legs during sleep, for example kicking the legs.
Tympanic membrane	The Tympanic membrane is a thin membrane that separates the external ear from the middle ear. Its function is to transmit sound from the air to the ossicles inside the middle ear.

Chapter 24. Older Adult,

Risk factor	A Risk factor is a variable associated with an increased risk of disease or infection. Risk factors are correlational and not necessarily causal, because correlation does not imply causation. For example, being young cannot be said to cause measles, but young people are more at risk as they are less likely to have developed immunity during a previous epidemic.
Decubitus ulcers	Bedsores, more properly known as pressure ulcers or Decubitus ulcers, are lesions caused by many factors such as: unrelieved pressure; friction; humidity; shearing forces; temperature; age; continence and medication; to any part of the body, especially portions over bony or cartilaginous areas such as sacrum, elbows, knees, ankles etc. Although easily prevented and completely treatable if found early, bedsores are often fatal - even under the auspices of medical care - and are one of the leading iatrogenic causes of death reported in developed countries, second only to adverse drug reactions. Prior to the 1950s, treatment was ineffective until Doreen Norton showed that the primary cure and treatment was to remove the pressure by turning the patient every two hours.
Life expectancy	Life expectancy is the average number of years of life remaining at a given age. The term is most often used in the human context, but used also in plant or animal ecology and the calculation is based on the analysis of life tables (also known as actuarial tables). The term may also be used in the context of manufactured objects although the related term shelf life is used for consumer products and the term mean time to breakdown (MTTB) is used in engineering literature.
Case study	A Case study is a research methodology common in social science. It is based on an in-depth investigation of a single individual, group, or event to explore causation in order to find underlying principles.
Geriatric depression	Geriatric depression is the prolonged occurrence of depression in elderly-aged people. A meta-analysis done by the University of Liverpool found a 3.86% prevalence rate of depressed elderly in The People's Republic of China, compared to a 12% prevalence in Western Europe. Factors for depression in Chinese elderly are affected by Chinese culture, social expectations, and living conditions.
Geriatric Depression Scale	The Geriatric Depression Scale is a 30-item self-report assessment used to identify depression in the elderly.
	The Geriatric Depression Scale questions are answered 'yes' or 'no', instead of a five-category response set. This simplicity enables the scale to be used with ill or moderately cognitively impaired individuals.
Depression	Depression is a state of low mood and aversion to activity that can affect a person's thoughts, behaviour, feelings and physical well-being. It may include feelings of sadness, anxiety, emptiness, hopelessness, worthlessness, guilt, irritability, or restlessness.

Euthanasia	Euthanasia) refers to the practice of ending a life in a painless manner. Many different forms of Euthanasia can be distinguished, including animal Euthanasia and human Euthanasia, and within the latter, voluntary and involuntary Euthanasia. Voluntary Euthanasia and physician-assisted suicide have been the focus of great controversy in recent years.
Osteoporosis	Osteoporosis is a disease of bones that leads to an increased risk of fracture. In osteoporosis the bone mineral density (BMD) is reduced, bone microarchitecture deteriorates, and the amount and variety of proteins in bone is altered. Osteoporosis is defined by the World Health Organization (WHO) as a bone mineral density that is 2.5 standard deviations or more below the mean peak bone mass (average of young, healthy adults) as measured by DXA; the term 'established osteoporosis' includes the presence of a fragility fracture.
Heat stroke	Heat stroke is defined as a temperature of greater than 40.6 °C (105.1 °F) due to environmental heat exposure with lack of thermoregulation. This is distinct from a fever, where there is a physiological increase in the temperature set point of the body. Treatment involves rapid mechanical cooling. A number of heat illnesses exist including: · Heat stroke as defined by a temperature of greater than >40.6 °C (105.1 °F) due to environmental heat exposure with lack of thermoregulation. · Heat exhaustion · Heat syncope · Heat edema · Heat cramps · Heat tetany Heat stroke presents with a hyperthermia of greater than >40.6 °C (105.1 °F) in combination with confusion and a lack of sweating.
Prevention	Prevention refers to: · Preventive medicine · Hazard Prevention, the process of risk study and elimination and mitigation in emergency management · Risk Prevention · Risk management · Preventive maintenance · Crime Prevention · Prevention, an album by Scottish band De Rosa · Prevention a magazine about health in the United States · Prevent (company), a textile company from Slovenia
Pneumococcal infection	Pneumococcal infection refers to an infection caused by Streptococcus pneumoniae. S. pneumoniae is normally found in the nasopharynx of 5-10% of healthy adults, and 20-40% of healthy children.

Chapter 24. Older Adult,

Alcohol abuse	Alcohol abuse, as described in the DSM-IV, is a psychiatric diagnosis describing the recurring use of alcoholic beverages despite negative consequences. It is differentiated from alcohol dependence by the lack of symptoms such as tolerance and withdrawal. Alcohol abuse is sometimes referred to by the less specific term alcoholism.
Prescription drug	A Prescription drug is a licensed medicine that is regulated by legislation to require a prescription before it can be obtained. The term is used to distinguish it from over-the-counter drugs which can be obtained without a prescription. Different jurisdictions have different definitions of what constitutes a Prescription drug.
Prostate cancer	Prostate cancer is a form of cancer that develops in the prostate, a gland in the male reproductive system. The cancer cells may metastasize (spread) from the prostate to other parts of the body, particularly the bones and lymph nodes. Prostate cancer may cause pain, difficulty in urinating, problems during sexual intercourse, or erectile dysfunction.
Cancer	Cancer (medical term: malignant neoplasm) is a class of diseases in which a group of cells display uncontrolled growth, invasion that intrudes upon and destroys adjacent tissues, and sometimes metastasis, or spreading to other locations in the body via lymph or blood. These three malignant properties of cancers differentiate them from benign tumors, which do not invade or metastasize. Researchers divide the causes of cancer into two groups: those with an environmental cause and those with a hereditary genetic cause.
Cancer screening	Cancer screening occurs for many type of cancer including breast, prostate, lung, and colorectal cancer. Cancer screening is an attempt to detect unsuspected cancers in an asymptomatic population. Screening tests suitable for large numbers of healthy people must be relatively affordable, safe, noninvasive procedures with acceptably low rates of false positive results. If signs of cancer are detected, more definitive and invasive follow up tests are performed to confirm the diagnosis.
Acute care	Acute care is necessary treatment of a disease for only a short period of time in which a patient is treated for a brief but severe episode of illness. Many hospitals are Acute care facilities with the goal of discharging the patient as soon as the patient is deemed healthy and stable, with appropriate discharge instructions. The term is generally associated with care rendered in an emergency department, ambulatory care clinic, or other short-term stay facility.

Palliative care	Palliative care is any form of medical care or treatment that concentrates on reducing the severity of disease symptoms, rather than striving to halt, delay, or reverse progression of the disease itself or provide a cure. The goal is to prevent and relieve suffering and to improve quality of life for people facing serious, complex illness. Non-hospice Palliative care is not dependent on prognosis and is offered in conjunction with curative and all other appropriate forms of medical treatment.
Home care	Home care, (commonly referred to as domiciliary care), is health care , it is also known as skilled care) or by family and friends (also known as caregivers, primary caregiver, or voluntary caregivers who give informal care). Often, the term Home care is used to distinguish non-medical care or custodial care, which is care that is provided by persons who are not nurses, doctors, or other licensed medical personnel, whereas the term home health care, refers to care that is provided by licensed personnel. 'Home care', 'home health care', 'in-Home care' are phrases that are used interchangeably in the United States to mean any type of care given to a person in their own home.
Continuing care	A Continuing care community is a type of retirement community where a number of aging care needs, from assisted living, independent living and nursing home care, may all be met in a single residence, whether apartment or enclosed unit. Typically, elderly candidates move into a continuing-care retirement community (Continuing careRC) while still living independently, with few health risks or healthcare needs, and will remain reside there until end of life. As patrons progress in age, and medical needs change, the level of nursing care and service increases proportionally in response.
Health care	Health care , refers to the treatment and management of illness, and the preservation of health through services offered by the medical, dental, complementary and alternative medicine, pharmaceutical, clinical laboratory sciences , nursing, and allied health professions. Health care embraces all the goods and services designed to promote health, including 'preventive, curative and palliative interventions, whether directed to individuals or to populations'. Before the term Health care became popular, English-speakers referred to medicine or to the health sector and spoke of the treatment and prevention of illness and disease.
Health insurance	Health insurance is insurance that pays for medical expenses. It is sometimes used more broadly to include insurance covering disability or long-term nursing or custodial care needs. It may be provided through a government-sponsored social insurance program, or from private insurance companies.

Chapter 24. Older Adult,

1. _____ , refers to the treatment and management of illness, and the preservation of health through services offered by the medical, dental, complementary and alternative medicine, pharmaceutical, clinical laboratory sciences , nursing, and allied health professions. _____ embraces all the goods and services designed to promote health, including 'preventive, curative and palliative interventions, whether directed to individuals or to populations'.

   Before the term _____ became popular, English-speakers referred to medicine or to the health sector and spoke of the treatment and prevention of illness and disease.

   a. Bacteriophage
   b. Ambulatory care
   c. Environmental medicine
   d. Health care

2. _____ is a diagnosis given to individuals who have cognitive impairments beyond that expected for their age and education, but that do not interfere significantly with their daily activities. It is considered to be the boundary or transitional stage between normal aging and dementia. Although _____ can present with a variety of symptoms, when memory loss is the predominant symptom it is termed 'amnestic _____' and is frequently seen as a risk factor for Alzheimer's disease.

   a. Mild cognitive impairment
   b. Maternal health
   c. Party and play
   d. Pelvic congestion syndrome

3. _____ is a form of urinary incontinence.

   _____ is involuntary loss of urine occurring for no apparent reason while suddenly feeling the need or urge to urinate.

   The most common cause of _____ is involuntary and inappropriate detrusor muscle contractions.

   a. Urge incontinence
   b. Achilles tendon
   c. Acute HIV infection
   d. Adenoviridae

4. . Bedsores, more properly known as pressure ulcers or _____, are lesions caused by many factors such as: unrelieved pressure; friction; humidity; shearing forces; temperature; age; continence and medication; to any part of the body, especially portions over bony or cartilaginous areas such as sacrum, elbows, knees, ankles etc. Although easily prevented and completely treatable if found early, bedsores are often fatal - even under the auspices of medical care - and are one of the leading iatrogenic causes of death reported in developed countries, second only to adverse drug reactions. Prior to the 1950s, treatment was ineffective until Doreen Norton showed that the primary cure and treatment was to remove the pressure by turning the patient every two hours.

   a. Dermatosis neglecta
   b. Decubitus ulcers

Chapter 24. Older Adult,

c. burn
d. Miliaria

5. _____ (medical term: malignant neoplasm) is a class of diseases in which a group of cells display uncontrolled growth, invasion that intrudes upon and destroys adjacent tissues, and sometimes metastasis, or spreading to other locations in the body via lymph or blood. These three malignant properties of _____s differentiate them from benign tumors, which do not invade or metastasize.

Researchers divide the causes of _____ into two groups: those with an environmental cause and those with a hereditary genetic cause.

a. Cancer
b. B-cell lymphoma
c. Basal-like carcinoma
d. Bladder cancer

1. d
2. a
3. a
4. b
5. a

You can take the complete Chapter Practice Test

for Chapter 24. Older Adult,
on all key terms, persons, places, and concepts.

Online 99 Cents

http://www.epub1625.32.20273.24.cram101.com/

Use www.Cram101.com for all your study needs

including Cram101's online interactive problem solving labs in

chemistry, statistics, mathematics, and more.

Chapter 25. Health Promotion in the Twenty-First Century

CHAPTER OUTLINE: KEY TERMS, PEOPLE, PLACES, CONCEPTS

	Health promotion
	Transtheoretical model
	Malnutrition
	Protein-energy malnutrition
	Case study
	Panton-Valentine leukocidin
	Severe acute respiratory syndrome
	Staphylococcus aureus
	Symptom
	Health care
	Life expectancy
	Risk factor
	Public health
	Data collection
	International Health
	Smallpox
	Health education
	Toilet training
	Therapeutic touch

CHAPTER OUTLINE: KEY TERMS, PEOPLE, PLACES, CONCEPTS

	Breast self-examination
	Prevention
	Cardiovascular disease
	Smoking cessation
	Prescription drug
	Genetic variation

CHAPTER HIGHLIGHTS & NOTES: KEY TERMS, PEOPLE, PLACES, CONCEPTS

Health promotion	Health promotion has been defined by the World Health Organization's 2005 Bangkok Charter for Health promotion in a Globalized World as 'the process of enabling people to increase control over their health and its determinants, and thereby improve their health'. The primary means of Health promotion occur through developing healthy public policy that addresses the prerequisities of health such as income, housing, food security, employment, and quality working conditions. There is a tendency among public health officials and governments -- and this is especially the case in liberal nations such as Canada and the USA -- to reduce Health promotion to health education and social marketing focused on changing behavioral risk factors.
Transtheoretical model	The Transtheoretical model in health psychology is intended to explain or predict a person's success or failure in achieving a proposed behavior change, such as developing different habits. It attempts to answer why the change 'stuck' or alternatively why the change was not made. The Transtheoretical model is also known by the acronym 'TTranstheoretical model' and by the term 'stages of change model'.
Malnutrition	Malnutrition is the insufficient, excessive or imbalanced consumption of nutrients. A number of different nutrition disorders may arise, depending on which nutrients are under or overabundant in the diet.

Chapter 25. Health Promotion in the Twenty-First Century

Protein-energy malnutrition	Protein-energy malnutrition refers to a form of malnutrition where there is inadequate protein intake. Types include: · Kwashiorkor (protein malnutrition predominant) · Marasmus (deficiency in both calorie and protein nutrition) · Marasmic Kwashiorkor (marked protein deficiency and marked calorie insufficiency signs present, sometimes referred to as the most severe form of malnutrition) Note that this may also be secondary to other conditions such as chronic renal disease or cancer cachexia in which protein energy wasting may occur. Protein-energy malnutrition effects children the most because they have less protein intake. The few rare cases found in the developed world are almost entirely found in small children as a result of fad diets, or ignorance of the nutritional needs of children, particularly in cases of milk allergy. · Bistrian BR, McCowen KC, Chan S (January 1999).
Case study	A Case study is a research methodology common in social science. It is based on an in-depth investigation of a single individual, group, or event to explore causation in order to find underlying principles.
Panton-Valentine leukocidin	Panton-Valentine leukocidin is a cytotoxin--one of the β-pore-forming toxins. The presence of Panton Valentine leukocidin is associated with increased virulence of certain strains (isolates) of Staphylococcus aureus. It is present in the majority of community-associated Methicillin-resistant Staphylococcus aureus (CA-MRSA) isolates studied and is the cause of necrotic lesions involving the skin or mucosa, including necrotic hemorrhagic pneumonia.
Severe acute respiratory syndrome	Severe acute respiratory syndrome is a respiratory disease in humans which is caused by the Severe acute respiratory syndrome coronavirus (Severe acute respiratory syndrome-CoV). There has been one near pandemic to date, between the months of November 2002 and July 2003, with 8,096 known infected cases and 774 confirmed human deaths (a case-fatality rate of 9.6%) worldwide being listed in the World Health Organization's (WHO) 21 April 2004 concluding report. Within a matter of weeks in early 2003, Severe acute respiratory syndrome spread from the Guangdong province of China to rapidly infect individuals in some 37 countries around the world.
Staphylococcus aureus	Staphylococcus aureus is a facultatively anaerobic, gram positive coccus and is the most common cause of staph infections. It is a spherical bacterium, frequently part of the skin flora found in the nose and on skin. About 20% of the population are long-term carriers of S.

Symptom	A symptom is a departure from normal function or feeling which is noticed by a patient, indicating the presence of disease or abnormality. A symptom is subjective, observed by the patient, and not measured. A symptom may not be a malady, for example symptoms of pregnancy.
Health care	Health care , refers to the treatment and management of illness, and the preservation of health through services offered by the medical, dental, complementary and alternative medicine, pharmaceutical, clinical laboratory sciences , nursing, and allied health professions. Health care embraces all the goods and services designed to promote health, including 'preventive, curative and palliative interventions, whether directed to individuals or to populations'. Before the term Health care became popular, English-speakers referred to medicine or to the health sector and spoke of the treatment and prevention of illness and disease.
Life expectancy	Life expectancy is the average number of years of life remaining at a given age. The term is most often used in the human context, but used also in plant or animal ecology and the calculation is based on the analysis of life tables (also known as actuarial tables). The term may also be used in the context of manufactured objects although the related term shelf life is used for consumer products and the term mean time to breakdown (MTTB) is used in engineering literature.
Risk factor	A Risk factor is a variable associated with an increased risk of disease or infection. Risk factors are correlational and not necessarily causal, because correlation does not imply causation. For example, being young cannot be said to cause measles, but young people are more at risk as they are less likely to have developed immunity during a previous epidemic.
Public health	Public health is 'the science and art of preventing disease, prolonging life and promoting health through the organized efforts and informed choices of society, organizations, public and private, communities and individuals.' (1920, C.E.A. Winslow) It is concerned with threats to the overall health of a community based on population health analysis. The population in question can be as small as a handful of people or as large as all the inhabitants of several continents (for instance, in the case of a pandemic). Public health is typically divided into epidemiology, biostatistics and health services.
Data collection	Data collection is a term used to describe a process of preparing and collecting data - for example as part of a process improvement or similar project. The purpose of Data collection is to obtain information to keep on record, to make decisions about important issues, to pass information on to others. Primarily, data is collected to provide information regarding a specific topic.

Chapter 25. Health Promotion in the Twenty-First Century

Data collection usually takes place early on in an improvement project, and is often formalised through a Data collection plan which often contains the following activity.

· Pre collection activity - Agree goals, target data, definitions, methods· Collection - Data collection· Present Findings - usually involves some form of sorting analysis and/or presentation.

International Health	International health, is a field of health care, usually with a public health emphasis, dealing with health across regional or national boundaries. One subset of international medicine, travel medicine, prepares travelers with immunizations, prophylactic medications, preventive techniques such as bednets and residual pesticides, in-transit care, and post-travel care for exotic illnesses. International health, however, more often refers to health personnel or organizations from one area or nation providing direct health care, or health sector development, in another area or nation.
Smallpox	Smallpox is an infectious disease unique to humans, caused by either of two virus variants, Variola major and Variola minor. The disease is also known by the Latin names Variola or Variola vera, which is a derivative of the Latin varius, meaning 'spotted', or varus, meaning 'pimple'. The term 'smallpox' was first used in Europe in the 15th century to distinguish variola from the 'great pox' (syphilis).
Health education	Health education is the profession of educating people about health. Areas within this profession encompass environmental health, physical health, social health, emotional health, intellectual health, and spiritual health. It can be defined as the principle by which individuals and groups of people learn to behave in a manner conducive to the promotion, maintenance, or restoration of health.
Toilet training	Toilet training, or potty training, is the process of training a young child to use the toilet for urination and defecation, though training may start with a smaller toilet bowl-shaped device (often known as a potty). In Western countries it is usually started and completed between the ages of 12 months and three years with boys typically being at the higher end of the age spectrum. Cultural factors play a large part in what age is deemed appropriate, with the age being generally later in America. Most advise that Toilet training is a mutual task, requiring cooperation, agreement and understanding between child and the caregiver, and the best potty training techniques emphasize consistency and positive reinforcement over punishment - making it fun for the child.

Therapeutic touch	Therapeutic touch (commonly shortened to),) or Distance Healing, is an energy therapy claimed to promote healing and reduce pain and anxiety. Practitioners of Therapeutic touch claim that by placing their hands on, or near, a patient, they are able to detect and manipulate the patient's putative energy field. Although there are currently (September 2009) 259 articles concerning Therapeutic touch on PubMed the quality of controlled research and tests is variable.
Breast self-examination	Breast self-examination (Breast self-examinationE) is a method of finding abnormalities of the breast, for early detection of breast cancer. The method involves the woman herself looking at and feeling each breast for possible lumps, distortions or swelling. Breast self-examinationE was once promoted heavily as a means of finding cancer at a more curable stage, but randomized controlled studies found that it was not effective in preventing death, and actually caused harm through needless biopsies and surgery.
Prevention	Prevention refers to: · Preventive medicine · Hazard Prevention, the process of risk study and elimination and mitigation in emergency management · Risk Prevention · Risk management · Preventive maintenance · Crime Prevention · Prevention, an album by Scottish band De Rosa · Prevention a magazine about health in the United States · Prevent (company), a textile company from Slovenia
Cardiovascular disease	Cardiovascular disease or Cardiovascular diseases refers to the class of diseases that involve the heart or blood vessels (arteries and veins). While the term technically refers to any disease that affects the cardiovascular system (as used in MeSH), it is usually used to refer to those related to atherosclerosis (arterial disease). These conditions have similar causes, mechanisms, and treatments.
Smoking cessation	Smoking cessation is the action leading towards the discontinuation of the consumption of a smoked substance, mainly tobacco, but it may encompass cannabis and other substances as well. Smoking certain substances can be addictive. This encompasses both psychological and biological addiction.
Prescription drug	A Prescription drug is a licensed medicine that is regulated by legislation to require a prescription before it can be obtained. The term is used to distinguish it from over-the-counter drugs which can be obtained without a prescription. Different jurisdictions have different definitions of what constitutes a Prescription drug.

Chapter 25. Health Promotion in the Twenty-First Century

Genetic variation	Genetic variation, variation in alleles of genes, occurs both within and among populations. Genetic variation is important because it provides the 'raw material' for natural selection. Genetic variation among individuals within a population can be identified at a variety of levels.

1. _____ or _____s refers to the class of diseases that involve the heart or blood vessels (arteries and veins). While the term technically refers to any disease that affects the cardiovascular system (as used in MeSH), it is usually used to refer to those related to atherosclerosis (arterial disease). These conditions have similar causes, mechanisms, and treatments.

   a. Bacteriophage
   b. Caliciviridae
   c. chromosome translocation
   d. Cardiovascular disease

2. The _____ in health psychology is intended to explain or predict a person's success or failure in achieving a proposed behavior change, such as developing different habits. It attempts to answer why the change 'stuck' or alternatively why the change was not made.

   The _____ is also known by the acronym 'TTranstheoretical model' and by the term 'stages of change model'.

   a. Bacteriophage
   b. Transtheoretical model
   c. Benign prostatic hyperplasia
   d. Benzathine benzylpenicillin

3. A _____ is a departure from normal function or feeling which is noticed by a patient, indicating the presence of disease or abnormality. A _____ is subjective, observed by the patient, and not measured.

   A _____ may not be a malady, for example _____s of pregnancy.

   a. Tachypnea
   b. Symptom
   c. Target lesion
   d. Tetanic contraction

4. _____ has been defined by the World Health Organization's 2005 Bangkok Charter for _____ in a Globalized World as 'the process of enabling people to increase control over their health and its determinants, and thereby improve their health'. The primary means of _____ occur through developing healthy public policy that addresses the prerequisities of health such as income, housing, food security, employment, and quality working conditions. There is a tendency among public health officials and governments -- and this is especially the case in liberal nations such as Canada and the USA -- to reduce _____ to health education and social marketing focused on changing behavioral risk factors.

a. Bacteriophage
b. Baroreflex
c. Health promotion
d. Benzathine benzylpenicillin

5. A _____ is a research methodology common in social science. It is based on an in-depth investigation of a single individual, group, or event to explore causation in order to find underlying principles.

a. Bacteriophage
b. Baroreflex
c. Case study
d. Benzathine benzylpenicillin

1. d
2. b
3. b
4. c
5. c

You can take the complete Chapter Practice Test

for Chapter 25. Health Promotion in the Twenty-First Century
on all key terms, persons, places, and concepts.

Online 99 Cents

http://www.epub1625.32.20273.25.cram101.com/

Use www.Cram101.com for all your study needs

including Cram101's online interactive problem solving labs in

chemistry, statistics, mathematics, and more.

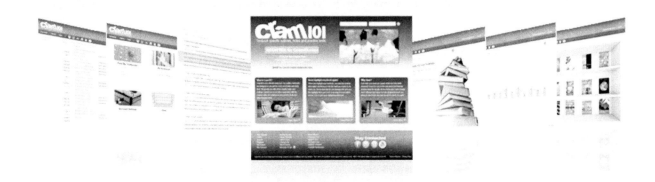

CPSIA information can be obtained at www.ICGtesting.com
Printed in the USA
LVOW090339150413

329146LV00001B/16/P